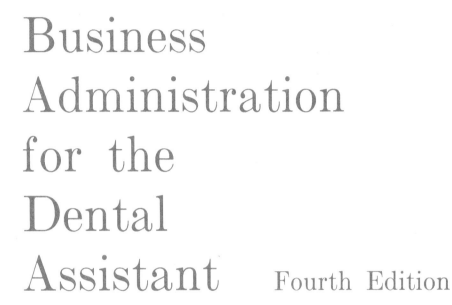

Business Administration for the Dental Assistant Fourth Edition

By Ann Ehrlich, M.A.

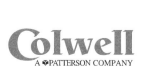

Colwell
A ❤ PATTERSON COMPANY

Published by
Colwell Systems
Champaign, Illinois 61820

Table of Contents

Chapter 1

ORIENTATION TO BUSINESS ADMINISTRATION

LEARNING GOALS

The student will be able to:

▶ Identify and describe at least three different roles within the business office.

▶ State why good communication skills are important in working with patients and fellow employees.

▶ Describe how to handle putting a patient on hold and managing a patient who insists upon speaking to the dentist.

▶ Identify the two forms of after hours telephone coverage and describe how to work with each.

▶ Demonstrate the proper method for answering the telephone and for taking messages.

▶ Demonstrate greeting practice visitors.

▶ Demonstrate completing a new patient registration and a medical and dental history form.

▶ Demonstrate handling a patient complaint.

2

OVERVIEW OF THE BUSINESS OFFICE

The business office is the control center of the dental practice. A well organized, efficient and smoothly functioning business office is an essential part of every successful practice. It is through the business office that:

- ✓ Telephone contact is established with new and returning patients.
- ✓ Patients are scheduled for treatment.
- ✓ Patients and visitors are greeted and made to feel welcome.
- ✓ Patient charts and records are maintained in an orderly manner so that they are protected and can be retrieved as necessary.
- ✓ Essential paperwork, such as insurance claims, financial records and government reports, are completed promptly and accurately.
- ✓ Accounts receivable records are maintained and money owed to the practice is collected.
- ✓ Practice expenses are managed in a business-like manner.

► Staffing Patterns

The staffing pattern of the dental business office depends upon the size of the practice and the doctor's specialty (Fig 1-1).

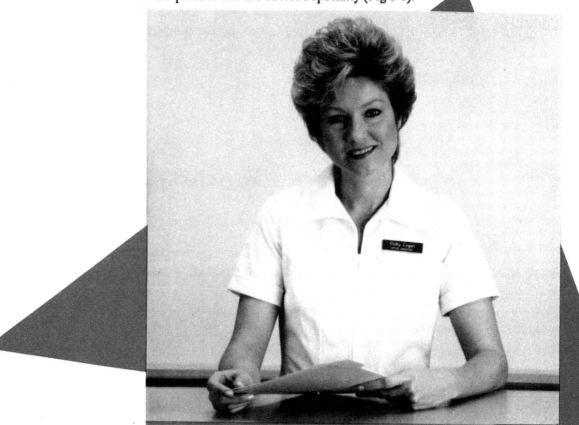

Figure 1-1. Your role in the business office is an important one!

In a solo practice, where the doctor works on long appointments and does not see a large volume of patients each day, a single secretarial assistant may be responsible for handling the entire business office.

In a busy group or specialty practice where a large number of patients are seen daily, there will be several workers in the business office, each with his or her own area of responsibility. For example, there may be one or more:

- **Receptionist(s)** — Who are responsible for answering the telephones, greeting practice visitors, typing and correspondence, and the smooth functioning of the reception area.
- **Appointments clerk(s)** — Who are responsible for all scheduling of patient visits. They also follow-up on broken appointments and manage rescheduling "changed appointment" times.
- **Insurance clerk(s)** — Who are responsible for completing, filing and following-up on all insurance claims and payments.
- **File clerk(s)** — Who are responsible for filing and retrieving patient records as needed.
- **Bookkeeper(s)** — Who are responsible for the management of all accounts receivable bookkeeping entries and records. The bookkeeper may also handle accounts payable bookkeeping.
- **Accounts receivable manager(s)** — Who are responsible for making financial arrangements with patients and for collecting all overdue accounts.
- **Office manager** — Who, in a very large practice, is responsible for the supervision of all business office activities.

In the "average practice" the staffing pattern generally includes two or three workers sharing all of these business office responsibilities.

▶ Your Role In The Business Office

Your role in the business office is an important one! By delegating these activities to you and other staff members, the dentist is able to concentrate on providing quality patient care. However, in doing this the dentist is placing great trust and confidence in you — any negligence on your part could affect the success of the entire practice (Fig 1-2).

In order to do your very best in this role, you need basic knowledge of the language of dentistry and the procedures being performed. In addition, you must also have the appropriate secretarial, business and communication skills.

Even if you plan to specialize in one area, such as insurance claims management, it is important that you learn the basics of *each* of the roles to be filled in the business office. Having this background knowledge will help you work more effectively with the other members of the office team.

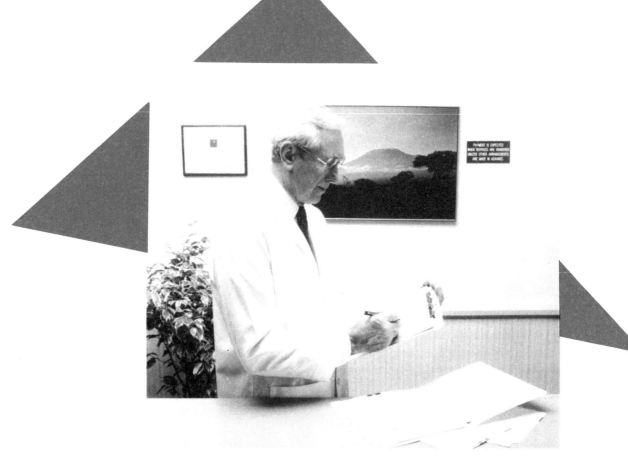

Figure 1-2. The dentist places great trust and confidence in the business office staff.

MANUAL AND COMPUTERIZED BUSINESS OFFICE SYSTEMS

In a solo or small dental group practice, all of the business office functions can be managed with very effective manual systems. However, in larger group practices some of these functions may be handled more efficiently with a computerized system.

Although computerized and manual systems seem very different, they really are not — for both require the same information. In fact, the only major difference is the manner in which information is recorded, stored and manipulated.

It is important that you learn the <u>basics</u> of each of the business office systems. With this understanding, you can then adapt easily to using either a manual or a computerized application.

Throughout this text, the basics of each system will be explained. Then, as appropriate, you will be shown how this works on either a manual or a computerized system.

BUILDING BETTER COMMUNICATION SKILLS

As you greet the public, you represent the dentist, the practice, and the profession of dentistry. It is through contact with you that the patient forms that very important first impression of the practice.

It is your professionalism, mixed with warmth and a genuine concern for people, that helps the new patient to be happy in the practice. And all of this happens before the patient has met the dentist!

▶ First impressions are lasting impressions.

Your appearance is important too. You should always be well-groomed and neatly uniformed. This includes a bright, sunny smile and a cheerful, cooperative attitude. By taking pride in yourself, you show admiration and respect for dentistry, your employer, and your profession.

Having good communication skills is important as you interact with patients and with your co-workers. A major part of building good communication skills is a willingness to understand how others are feeling and a genuine desire to help them.

▶ Keys To Good Listening

Listening is not a passive activity — or a natural skill. It is something that all of us must really work at if we are to do it successfully. The steps to becoming a better listener are outlined in the Table *"Steps To Becoming A Better Listener."*

STEPS TO BECOMING A BETTER LISTENER	
DO...	**DON'T...**
● **Limit your own talking.** You can't talk and listen at the same time. You can learn a lot more by listening.	● **Interrupt.** It is common courtesy to let the patient finish the explanation before you jump in with your next remark or suggestion.
● **Listen for more than words.** Make an effort to listen for the emotions behind the words. Often these feelings are an important clue to what the patient is really feeling and trying to express!	● **Argue.** Try to be understanding and accepting of what the patient is saying (even if you don't agree).
● **Think like the patient.** The patient's problems and needs are important. You'll understand what is being said better if you try to see the situation from the patient's point of view.	● **Be pushy.** Don't try to force your point of view on the patient.
● **Concentrate on listening.** You can't listen effectively if you are busy formulating your reply or wondering what you are going to have for lunch.	● **Jump to conclusions.** If you aren't sure about what the patient said, ask clarifying questions.

▶ Asking Questions

We all use questions to gather information; however, the way you phrase a question determines the kind of answer you get. By being aware of this, you can more effectively gather information and help the patients feel at ease.

Closed-Ended Questions

A closed-ended question is one which can be answered "yes" or "no." These questions are best used to confirm information, to limit a conversation or to close a conversation.

Closed-ended questions often begin with the words *IS, DO, HAS, CAN, WILL* or *SHALL.*

For example, "*Mrs. Andrews, IS Tuesday at 2 P.M. convenient for you?*" is a closed-ended question that can only be answered "yes" or "no."

Open-Ended Questions

An open-ended question is one which requires more than a "yes" or "no" answer. These questions are best used when you want to obtain information, maintain control of the conversation, or build rapport. (**Rapport** is a feeling of harmony and accord.)

Open-ended questions usually begin with the words *WHAT, WHEN, HOW, WHO, WHERE* or *WHICH.*

For example, "*Mr. Riccardo, WHAT time of day is best to schedule your appointment?*" is an open-ended question.

▶ Words Are Important

Words can hurt, and your choice of words in talking with patients is important. If you use technical terms when they aren't really necessary, you may confuse the listener.

There are also emotionally loaded words, such as *pain* or *pull,* that are best avoided because they can increase the patient's uneasiness and anxiety. The words in the Table "*Finding The Better Word*" are examples of how you can show your concern for the patient by selecting your words very carefully.

GREETING PRACTICE VISITORS

The reception area and business office should be kept neat and clean at all times. If the arriving visitor sees dying plants or drooping flowers, torn magazines strewn about or toys underfoot, he may well wonder whether or not anyone in the practice is concerned about sanitary conditions and quality care.

▶ Everyone who enters the reception area should be greeted promptly and pleasantly.

Everyone who enters the reception area should be greeted <u>promptly</u> and <u>pleasantly</u>. Before going into the reception area to greet the new arrival, check the appointment book to see which patient is due to arrive next. (Having this information will give you a head start on being able to greet the visitor by name.)

If you do not know the waiting visitor, introduce yourself and then tactfully ask the caller's name and reason for coming.

FINDING THE BETTER WORD	
Instead of this . . .	**Say this . . .**
Waiting room	Reception area
Pain	Discomfort
Pull	Remove
Filling	Restoration
False teeth	Denture
Bill	Statement
Operatory	Treatment room
Drill or grind	Prepare the tooth
Acid etch	Condition

▶ Addressing The Patient Properly

As a way of showing respect, all adults should be addressed as *"Mr. Jones," "Mrs. Smith,"* or *"Miss Thomas"* and not by their first name.

Of course, if the patient says, *"Oh, please call me George,"* then you would honor this request (and make a note of it on the patient's chart).

▶ Greeting Patient With Appointments

If the caller is a patient with an appointment, it is courteous to mention how long the wait will be. If the patient must wait because an emergency has disrupted the schedule, apologize for the delay and explain that the doctor has been delayed by an "emergency." (It is not necessary to provide any further details of the emergency.)

▶ Greeting Callers Without Appointments

If the caller is not a patient with an appointment, find out the reason for the call so that you can handle this visit appropriately.

For example, if the caller is a sales representative, follow the doctor's policy as to when these representatives are to be seen. If the doctor cannot see the caller, indicate this politely but firmly.

If the caller is a patient without an appointment, this too is handled according to the doctor's policy. ("Walk-in patients" are discussed in Chapter 2, Scheduling and Appointment Control.)

NEW PATIENT "PAPER WORK"

It is necessary to gather basic information from all new patients. This usually includes a patient registration form (for financial data) and a medical and dental history (for clinical data).

A new patient should be asked to come to the first appointment a few minutes early so that these forms can be completed before the patient is seen by the dentist.

When a patient returns, for example at a recall visit, verify that the information on these forms is still accurate.

▶ The Patient Registration Form

New patients should be asked to complete a patient registration form such as the one shown in Figure 1-3.

These forms are used to gather basic financial background and account identification information for the entire patient family.

If a family member has already completed one of these forms, it is only necessary to see that the data for the new patient is included on that form.

Section #1

The first section of the form gathers data regarding the person responsible for the account. This information will be used in the accounts receivable bookkeeping to maintain billing records and in preparing insurance claims.

Many registration forms ask for *the name and address of nearest relative not living with you.* This is called the **secondary address** and is used in case of emergency.

This information may also be necessary if a patient moves without having paid the bill — or leaving a forwarding address.

Many practices also request the **referral source.** Referrals are very important to the practice growth and this information may be used so that the doctor can acknowledge the referral.

Section #2

The second section gathers specific information for <u>each</u> family member. This information is used primarily in preparing insurance claims.

Section #3

The third section gathers data concerning the family's insurance coverage. It is necessary to gather this information for each family member who is employed and has insurance coverage.

Storing Patient Registration Forms

Since patient registration records are not clinical records, they should not be filed with the patient's chart. The patient registration form shown in Figure 1-3 is provided three-hole punched so that these forms can be filed alphabetically in a three-ring binder. This binder is stored in the business office where it can be used for reference as necessary.

PATIENT REGISTRATION FORM

Responsible Party __James_____A._____Gridley_____
                      First Name   Initial   Last Name

Address ___670 Northridge Terrace_____

_____

City ___Champaign_____ State _____IL_____ Zip Code ___61820_____

Phone: (Home)___351-4498_____ (Work)___322-0987_____

Employer ___Champion Automotive Supply_____

Address ___9000 Broad Street, Champaign, IL 61820_____

Name & Address of Nearest Relative (not living with you)_____

_____ Phone _____

Referral Source ___Grace Hardy_____

Family Member Information

	First Name	Last Name	Sex	Relationship* I–S–C–O	Birthday
Pt. #					
(1)	James	Gridley	M	I	04/05/55
(2)	Ruth	Gridley	F	S	11/30/56
(3)	Lisa	Gridley	F	C	06/20/83
(4)	Ben	Gridley	M	C	10/01/85

Please list additional members on reverse.   *I = Insured, S = Spouse, C = Child, O = Other Dependent

Dental Insurance Information

Subscriber Name___James A. Gridley_____ S.S. #___890-49-5381_____ Pt. #___1___

Carrier Name & Address ___Equitable_____

___2000 Tower Place, New York, NY 10003_____

Group Name___Champion Auto_____ Group Number___CH-23000_____

Does this plan cover all family members? __XX__Yes ___No

If no specify those **NOT** Covered.

ASSIGNMENT OF BENEFITS	**RELEASE OF INFORMATION**
I authorize payment of dental benefits to myself or the named provider for professional services rendered.	I authorize the release of any dental information necessary to process this claim.
Signed _James A. Gridley_ Date_1/9/xx_ (Subscriber)	Signed _James A. Gridley_ Date_1/9/xx_ (Patient, or parent if Minor)

Figure 1-3. Patient registration form sample.

▶ The Medical And Dental History

The patient should also be asked to complete a medical and dental history form such as the one shown in Figure 1-4. In some practices, this is done in the reception area before the patient sees the dentist. In other practices, the dentist or assistant goes over this form with the patient in the treatment area.

A single patient registration form is completed for the entire family. However, each new patient must complete an individual medical and dental history. This is clinical information which becomes part of the patient's clinical record.

▶ The Welcome Brochure

Just as the practice needs to gather patient data, the patient wants information about the practice. This is provided to the patient in the form of a welcome brochure (Fig 1-5).

This brochure contains helpful information about: office hours, emergency care, telephone calls, fees and payments, and insurance.

When giving the brochure to the patient, you might say, "*This is information about the practice that doctor thought would be important to you. If you have any other questions, please feel free to ask.*"

THE TELEPHONE

▶ Telephone calls are not an interruption, they are an important part of your job!

The telephone is a major source of contact with both new and returning patients. Therefore, it is important to remember that telephone calls are not an interruption, they are an essential part of your job!

You are responsible for answering the phone in a manner that creates a favorable impression and allows you to handle calls efficiently. When talking face-to-face with someone, your smile, appearance and warmth combine to create a good impression. However, when you speak over the telephone, everything depends on your voice.

If you are tired, bored or rushed, these negative feelings will be evident in your voice. You don't want to let this happen. Instead, make an effort to have your voice convey enthusiasm, interest and concern for the caller.

Also, never eat, drink or chew gum while talking on the telephone. Instead, speak slowly and clearly into the telephone and give the caller your full attention.

▶ Using The Proper Greeting

As you answer the telephone, take a deep breath, relax and smile. Then use the greeting that is preferred by your employer. Generally this includes:

- **The greeting.** This should be either "*Good morning*" or "*Good afternoon.*"
- **Identify the practice.** This should be either the name of the dentist or of the practice. For example, "*Dr. Taylor's office,*" or "*Urbana Dental Group.*"

Date _____

Name _Harriet Barnes_   Date of Birth _2/28/60_

Address _2951 Broadview Terrace, Champaign, Il_   Telephone _351-0241_

Business Address _____   Business Phone _____

Soc. Sec. No. _140-20-9123_

PATIENT MEDICAL HISTORY

Physician _Henry Thomas_   Office Phone _352-2043_   Home Phone _____

Approximate date of last physical examination _2 yrs._

		Yes	No
1.	Are you under any medical treatment now?	☐	☑
2.	Have you had any major operations? If so what? _appendectomy_	☑	☐
3.	Have you ever had a serious accident involving head injuries?	☐	☑
4.	Have you had any adverse response to any drugs including penicillin? _penicillin_	☑	☐
5.	Has a physician ever informed you that you had: A Heart Ailment?	☐	☑
6.	High Blood Pressure?	☐	☑
7.	Respiratory Disease?	☐	☑
8.	Diabetes?	☐	☑
9.	Rheumatic Fever?	☐	☑
10.	Rheumatism or Arthritis?	☐	☑
11.	Tumors or Growths	☐	☑
12.	Any Blood Disease?	☐	☑
13.	Any Liver Disease?	☐	☑
14.	Any Kidney Disease?	☐	☑
15.	Any Stomach or Intestinal Disease?	☐	☑
16.	Any Venereal Disease?	☐	☑
17.	AIDS?	☐	☑
18.	Yellow Jaundice or Hepatitis?	☐	☑
19.	Do you have night sweats accompanied by weight loss or cough?	☐	☑
20.	Are you on a diet at this time?	☑	☐
21.	Are you now taking drugs or medications?	☐	☑
22.	Are you allergic to any known materials resulting in hives, asthma, eczema, etc.?	☐	☑
23.	Are you in general good health at this time?	☑	☐
24.	Have any wounds healed slowly or presented other complications?	☐	☑
25.	Are you pregnant?	☐	☑
26.	Do you have a history of fainting?	☐	☑
27.	Have you ever had any X-RAY TREATMENTS (other than diagnostic)?	☐	☑

PATIENT DENTAL HISTORY

		Yes	No
28.	Do you have pain in or near your ears?	☐	☑
29.	Do you have any unhealed injuries or inflamed areas in or around your mouth?	☐	☑
30.	Have you experienced any growth or sore spots in your mouth?	☐	☑
31.	Does any part of your mouth hurt when clenched?	☑	☐
32.	Have you ever had Novocaine anesthetic?	☑	☐
33.	Any reactions or allergic symptoms to Novocaine?	☐	☑
34.	Any difficult extractions in the past?	☐	☑
35.	Prolonged bleeding following extractions in the past?	☐	☑
36.	Trench Mouth?	☐	☑
37.	Do your gums bleed?	☐	☑
38.	Have you ever had instruction on the correct method of brushing your teeth?	☑	☐
39.	Have you ever had instructions on the care of your gums?	☑	☐
40.	Do you chew on only one side of your mouth? If so why?	☐	☑
41.	Do you at the present time have any dental complaints?	☐	☑
42.	Do you habitually clench your teeth during the night or day?	☑	☐
43.	When was your last full mouth X-RAY taken? _1 year_ Where? _Seattle, WA_		
44.	Any part of your mouth sore to pressures or irritants (cold, sweets, etc.)	☐	☑
	If so locate _____		

Figure 1-4. Patient medical and dental history form sample.   Signature _Harriet Barnes_

FORM 9879 COLWELL SYSTEMS, INC., CHAMPAIGN, IL 61820

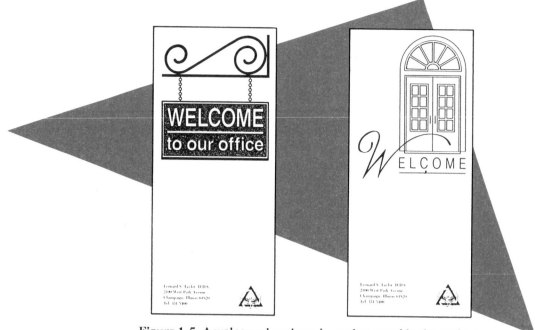

Figure 1-5. A welcome brochure is used to provide the patient with information about the practice.

- **Identify yourself.** It is important that you let the caller know who you are; however, it is not necessary to give your full name. For example, *"This is Sue speaking."* is acceptable.
- **Offer to help.** By asking, *"How may I help you?"* This lets the caller know that you want to help. It also discourages callers from asking to speak to the doctor.

The first step in the call itself is to find out who is calling and the reason for the call. Usually, after you have introduced yourself, the caller will respond with his or her name. If the caller doesn't, politely ask, *"Who is calling please?"* and then use the caller's name in the conversation.

As the caller explains the reason for the call, ask appropriate questions and make the notes you'll need to follow up on the call.

Terminate the conversation politely. It is courteous to thank the person for calling and to let the caller hang up first. When finished with the call, be sure to take any necessary follow-through action promptly.

► The Telephone Log

Many practices routinely enter all incoming calls in a telephone log or on a duplicate telephone message form (Fig 1-6). This creates a valuable office record which can be used to make certain that all inquiries and requests have been handled correctly.

► Placing The Caller On Hold

It is best to avoid putting the caller on hold. However, if you must put him on hold, always ask his permission first — and <u>wait</u> for him to respond before doing so.

Then, get back to the caller as quickly as possible. If the holding period is extended, inform caller of the wait and offer to return the call.

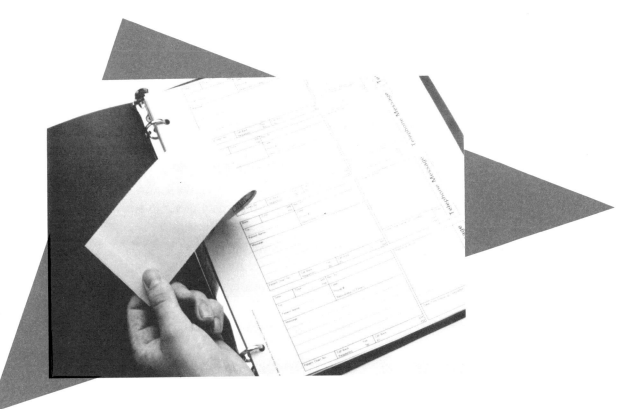

Figure 1-6. Telephone messages are taken in duplicate. The original is used to convey the message, the copy remains in the phone log.

The Routing Guide

The dentist should provide guidelines, in the form of a routing guide, as to how different types of calls are to be handled. For example questions regarding insurance claims go to the insurance clerk and appointment requests or scheduling changes go to the appointments clerk.

An important part of the guide should be instructions on how to handle emergency calls. Helpful questions to ask the caller, and the procedure for scheduling emergency patients, are discussed in Chapter 2.

The dentist is generally not available to come to the phone, and another important part of the routing guide is a list of the exceptions to this rule. Usually the dentist will include speaking to a:

- laboratory technician
- physician
- another dentist
- immediate family member

All other callers should be politely informed that, *"The dentist is with a patient now. May I help you, or would you like me to take a message so that the dentist can return your call?"* This should discourage the caller from insisting upon speaking to the dentist immediately.

The Patient Who Insists Upon Speaking To The Dentist

Despite this, some patients still insist upon speaking to the dentist. These callers are usually patients who are upset about something, and they present a difficult dilemma for you. After all, you don't want to interrupt the dentist — and you don't want to further upset the patient.

Before you are faced with this problem, ask the dentist how such a situation should be handled. (Many dentists would prefer to take such a phone call immediately — rather than risk further upsetting the patient.)

Then, when faced with the problem, you should stay calm and polite, express your concern and handle the call according to the dentist's instructions. After you hang up, carefully document the conversation in the telephone log.

If the patient does not speak to the dentist, and does not leave a message, it is a good idea to inform the dentist of the conversation. This will alert the dentist to a potential problem.

Taking Messages

If a message is taken, it is recorded in duplicate. The copy remains as part of the telephone log. The original is given to the doctor or appropriate person for follow-up action.

When taking a message, it is important that you gather all of the necessary information and record it accurately (Fig 1-7). This includes:

- ✓ Who called?
- ✓ When?
- ✓ Why?
- ✓ Is the call to be returned?
- ✓ If so, what is the phone number and who is to return the call?

If the dentist must return a call to a patient about a clinical question, pull that patient's chart and give it to the doctor along with the message. After the follow-up has been taken on this message, the action is noted on the form and the completed message form is filed in the patient's chart.

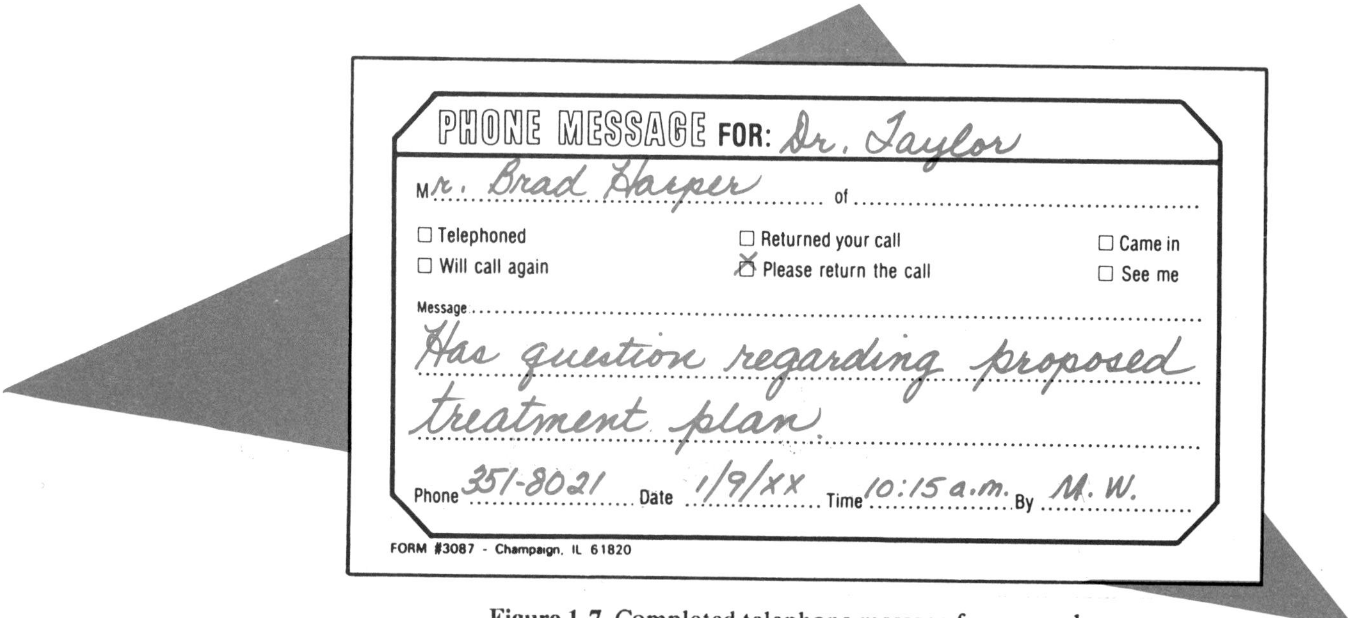
PHONE MESSAGE FOR: Dr. Taylor

Mr. Brad Harper of

☐ Telephoned ☐ Returned your call ☐ Came in

☐ Will call again ☒ Please return the call ☐ See me

Message

Has question regarding proposed treatment plan.

Phone 351-8021 Date 1/9/xx Time 10:15 a.m. By M. W.

FORM #3087 - Champaign, IL 61820

Figure 1-7. Completed telephone message form sample.

▶ After Hours Telephone Coverage

Some form of telephone coverage must be provided for those times when the office is closed. This is usually in the form of a telephone answering service or an answering machine.

The Answering Service

With an answering service, an operator answers the calls and handles them by either taking a message, paging the doctor, or forwarding the call.

Depending upon the arrangement, the service will answer when notified that calls are being forwarded to them or if the phone hasn't been answered after a certain number of rings. Either way, before the office is closed it is important to provide the service with this information:

- The day and time when the office will reopen.
- Whom to contact, and where to contact them, in case of an emergency.

When the office does reopen, notify the service immediately that you are back to receive any messages. As the messages are dictated, record them accurately and return these calls promptly.

The Answering Machine

After hours coverage may be provided by an answering machine located in the dental office.

When the office is closing, check that the machine is turned on and that it has the appropriate message. This message should tell the caller:

- The name of the office.
- How to reach the doctor in case of an emergency.
- How to leave a message for non-emergency calls.
- The office's call back policy.

Although it is helpful to the caller to know when the office will reopen, some doctors feel that this information might be useful to someone planning to break into the office. Therefore, data about the reopening day and time should be included only if this is the doctor's policy.

When the office reopens, check the machine immediately. Note the messages and double check them for accuracy, then erase the tape. Return the calls promptly.

▶ Personal Phone Calls

A dental practice is a business, and the phone lines are for business purposes. Also, the staff members all have responsibilities to carry out. For these reasons, staff members are asked to limit their use of the phones for personal calls.

In many practices, when a personal call is received for a staff member, the receptionist takes a message and has the call returned during lunch hour or on a break. (Obviously an emergency call would be an exception to this policy.)

HANDLING COMPLAINTS

Handling complaints is no fun. However, the following steps will help you handle these calls more easily and more effectively.

▶ You Are Not The Target

Except in unusual situations, the caller's complaint and anger are not directed at you. Keep in mind that you are not the target and remain calm no matter how upset the caller may be.

▶ Listen Without Interruption

While listening carefully, mentally sort through what the caller is saying. Your goal is to separate the actual complaint from any excessive elements such as sarcasm or exaggeration. Taking notes will help you concentrate on the "business part" of the call and ignore the obviously emotional or irrational parts.

▶ Express Your Regret

Regardless of whether or not you feel the complaint is justified, you should show sincere concern in your first statement to the caller. For example, you might say *"Mr. Higgins, I'm very sorry about the misunderstanding."*

▶ Restate The Complaint

Maintain your warmth and composure as you restate the complaint as you now understand it. Your goal is to try to get the caller to agree upon exactly what his complaint is. After all, you can't help with the complaint until you know what it is.

For example, *"Mr. Higgins, let me be sure that I understand. You feel that your statement shows charges for a visit that you don't remember making last month. Is that correct?"*

▶ Ask Questions

Rather than asking the caller to repeat the story (which usually will only increase his anger), ask open-ended questions as a means of gathering more information.

These logical questions tend to have a calming effect on the caller, and they allow you to gain control of the conversation.

▶ Assure Action

You may not have the answer to the caller's complaint; however, you can promise some form of action. For example you might say, *"Mr. Higgins, I'll go over your account and check our other records. Then, I'll call you back before five o'clock this afternoon."*

If you promise to call back, do it — even if you have to say that you are still working on the situation.

If possible, offer several options. This gives the caller a feeling of being a partner in resolving the problem. For example, "*Mr. Higgins, would you like me to call you back this afternoon, or would you prefer that I mail you a corrected statement?*"

When You Reach A Solution

Clarify your agreement with the caller so that you both are sure you understand the solution.

Follow Through

If you have promised to take additional action, be certain that you meet this commitment promptly so that the problem is resolved as promised.

Chapter

SCHEDULING AND APPOINTMENT CONTROL

LEARNING GOALS

The student will be able to:

▶ Name at least three key factors in appointment book selection.

▶ Describe the four steps in outlining the appointment book.

▶ List the basic rules for all appointment book entries, and identify the sequence in which these entries should be made.

▶ Discuss how to schedule appointments for emergency patients, walk-ins, recall patients, children and elderly patients.

▶ Describe how to maintain a system to reschedule changed appointment times.

▶ Discuss the functions of the daily schedule and describe where it should be posted.

▶ Identify the records that should be gathered in preparation for the patient's visit.

▶ Demonstrate making appointment book entries.

▶ Demonstrate completing appointment card entries.

OVERVIEW OF SCHEDULING AND APPOINTMENT CONTROL

A crowded reception room is <u>not</u> a sign of success!

There was a time when a crowded reception room was a sign of a busy doctor and a successful practice. This is no longer true. Today patients are not willing to wait endlessly. For most patients 15 minutes is an acceptable wait. Beyond this they become angry and impatient because they feel that the doctor has failed to recognize that their time is important too!

With good appointment management, the patients are scheduled efficiently and the work day runs smoothly with a well-balanced patient load. This enables the dentist to provide better care for more patients, while working with minimal stress.

When there are several staff members working in the business office, it is best to have <u>one</u> person responsible for all appointment planning and appointment book entries.

COMPUTERIZED APPOINTMENT CONTROL

Computerized scheduling and appointment control has the advantages of making it easier and faster to:

- Search for available time.
- Look up an appointment in response to a patient inquiry.
- Generate and revise a printed daily schedule.

However, the computerized scheduling system must be matrixed with the same information that is needed to outline in the appointment book. It is also still necessary that the appointment clerk have the information and skills necessary to plan and schedule appointments to assure a smooth flow of patients throughout the day.

With a fully computerized system, no paper appointment book is maintained. As a precaution, it is advisable to print daily schedules for several days in advance. Then, if the computer is down, these schedules may be used as a temporary appointment book while the system is being repaired.

APPOINTMENT BOOK SELECTION

The appointment book is one of the most important, and least expensive, tools used in the business office.

✓ The **right appointment book** helps to assure a smooth and efficient patient flow.

✓ The **wrong appointment book** may contribute to costly scheduling mix-ups and wasted time.

It is important that the practice be controlled through the appointment book — not by it.

Although the appointment book is the control center of the dental practice, it is important that the practice be controlled through it — but not by it.

There are many styles of appointment books available to choose from to fill the special needs of the practice. If a preprinted book does not fit these needs, it is possible to design your own through a custom printing service. When selecting an appointment book, the following important factors must be considered.

▶ Essential Information Per Patient Visit

The essential information to be listed for each patient visit is determined by the dentist. However because of the space limitations, it is necessary to restrict this to only the essentials. For most practices this includes:

- The patient's full name.
- Telephone numbers at home and work (for the confirmation call and in case it is necessary to change the schedule).
- A code to indicate the reason for the visit.

Figure 2-1 is a sample appointment book page. The codes used to indicate the procedures planned for each patient visit are explained in the Table *"Sample Reason For Visit Codes."*

▶ Overall Size

When deciding on the size of the book, it is important to remember that no matter how much space there is in the appointment book, the dentist can only be in one place at a time.

The overall size of the appointment book selected is usually a compromise between the amount of space needed for each appointment entry and the amount of desk space available to use the appointment book when it is *OPEN*.

When desk space is a problem, a wirebound book has the advantage that it may be used when folded back upon itself to save room. These books are available in the following sizes:

- A **regular size** wirebound appointment book is 9 x 22-7/8 inches when fully open and only 9 x 12 inches when folded back on itself.
- A **mid-size** appointment book is 11 x 26 inches when fully open and only 11 x 12-1/2 inches when folded back on itself.
- A **jumbo size** appointment book is 11 x 35-1/4 inches when fully open and only 11 x 17 inches when folded back on itself.

▶ Binding Styles

Appointment books are available in three different binding styles. These are hardbound, for use in a small practice where few patients are seen each day, or wirebound and looseleaf which are well suited for larger practices.

> ▶ No matter how much space there is in the appointment book, the dentist can only be in one place at a time.

SAMPLE REASON FOR VISIT CODES		
ca = corrective appliance	**ds** = denture service	**rc** = recall
c & b = crown and bridge	**ft** = fluoride treatment	**rct** = root canal therapy
co = consultation	**gt** = gingival treatment	**rests** = restorations
comp = composite restorations	**np** = new patient	**sr** = silver restoration
crown = crown preparation	**pot** = post operative treatment	**veneers** = cosmetic veneers

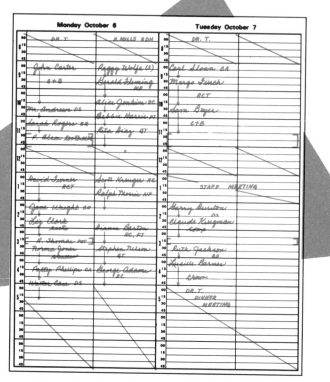

Figure 2-1. Sample appointment book page.

A **hardbound** appointment book has a cover like a hardback book. This style has the disadvantages that it does not lie flat on the desk, will not stay open to one page and is awkward to use when making entries.

A **wirebound** appointment book has the advantages that it is flexible in use, will lie flat on the desk, and can be folded back on itself to save space (Fig. 2-2).

A **looseleaf** appointment book has the advantage that pages can be added and removed as necessary (Fig. 2-3). This saves the wear and tear of having to sort through pages that are no longer in use. It also makes it possible to add pages for the new year without the necessity of having two appointment books in use at one time.

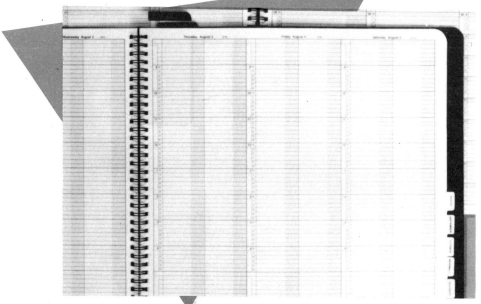

Figure 2-2. A wirebound appointment book is flexible in use and can be folded back on itself to save space.

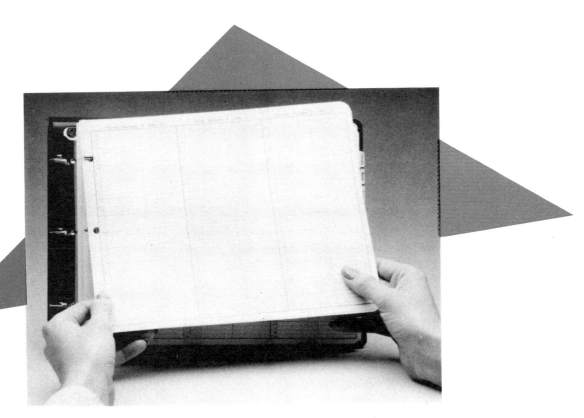

Figure 2-3. Looseleaf appointment book pages may be added or removed as necessary.

The most commonly used format for wirebound and looseleaf appointment books is a **week-in-view** with three days shown on each page. When the book is open, it is possible to review the schedule for an entire week at one glance.

▶ Number Of Columns Per Day

There must be enough space so that each entry will be easy to read and yet be complete with all necessary information about that appointment.

The space in the appointment book day is divided into two or three columns per day. These columns may be used in any one of these ways:

✓ Provide ample space to enter information concerning each scheduled patient.

✓ Schedule "by the operatory," using one column for each treatment room that will be in use at that time.

✓ Allow one column per provider. This makes it possible to maintain more than one schedule in a single appointment book. (In a dental practice a **provider** is a dentist or hygienist who maintains his or her own appointment schedule.)

▶ Units Of Time

Within the appointment book, each hour is divided into 10 or 15-minute units of time. The length of the time unit is determined by the dentist's preference. Most general practitioners work on 15-minute units; however, orthodontists favor the 10-minute units.

The time unit selected becomes the basis for the length of time that a patient will be scheduled. The number of units the dentist requests to be reserved for a patient will be based upon the treatment planned.

For example, Dr. Taylor works in 15-minute units and he is planning a bridge preparation for Harold Foster. Dr. Taylor requests that you reserve 4 time units for Mr. Foster.

This means that Mr. Foster's appointment will be sixty-minutes long. If Dr. Taylor were using 10-minute units, he would have requested that 6 time units be reserved for that appointment.

▶ Cover Colors

Appointment books are available in a wide range of colors which can be selected to blend with the office decor or other color preference.

Some group practices maintain a separate appointment book for each dentist. In this situation, having different cover colors makes it possible to quickly select the correct book.

▶ Dated And Undated Appointment Books

Appointment books are available in both dated and undated formats.

- A **dated appointment book** has the convenience of having the day and date already printed at the top of the columns for each day.
- An **undated appointment book** has space at the top of each day where the date can be written in.

An undated appointment book is well suited for a satellite office where patients are seen only a few days each week. This type of book also works well in a very large group practice where several pages are needed for each day.

▶ Dividers And Bookmarks

It is very convenient to have monthly index tabs to enable the user to turn quickly to the correct month (Fig 2-4).

Some dated appointment books come with these tabs already in place on the edge of the page.

With a looseleaf book, a monthly index (similar to notebook dividers) may be added to the book.

Another time saving idea is having a bookmark to indicate the current week. This might be a "*This week*" marker that slips on the binding of the wirebound appointment book. An alternative is to use a removable "tape flag" to indicate the current week.

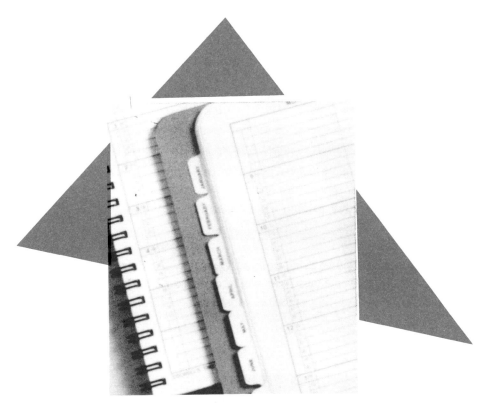

Figure 2-4. Monthly dividers speed finding the correct month in the appointment book.

OUTLINING THE APPOINTMENT BOOK

It is necessary to go through the appointment book well in advance and outline certain standard information. This is also called **matrixing** or **outlining** the book and it establishes the format of the days to come.

These outlining entries should be made in pencil that is dark enough to be seen easily — but erasable in case there is a change of plans. This information includes four elements:

#1 — Routine Hours

The times when the office is normally closed should be crossed out in the appointment book. These times include:

- Major holidays when the office is closed.
- The usual day(s) off during the week.
- Those hours shown in the appointment book before and after the office is open each day.
- Lunch hour for each provider.

#2 — Buffer Periods

Buffer periods are those times reserved each day for scheduling emergency patients. A buffer period is usually planned for one or two time units in late morning and one in the afternoon.

Buffer periods are indicated by brackets at the side of the reserved time. Since these times are saved so that emergency patients can be seen as soon as possible, the buffer periods are <u>not</u> filled more than a day in advance.

#3 — Meetings And Vacations

These are times reserved for staff meetings, educational programs and other occasions when the dentist must be out of the office.

Vacation time when the dentist or other provider will be away should be blocked out as soon as this information becomes available. (This will save having to reschedule patients when the dentist wants to go on vacation.)

#4 — Minor Holidays

A note should be made of minor holidays when the office will be open but schools and some businesses will be closed. Such times will be more convenient for scheduling school children and certain workers who may have the day off.

RULES FOR APPOINTMENT BOOK ENTRIES

▶ All appointment book entries must be legible, complete and in pencil.

These rules apply to all appointment book entries!

1. Do not use the appointment book as a social calendar.
   It is reserved only for scheduling entries.

2. All entries must be:
   * **Legible**
   * **Complete**
   * **In pencil**

3. Enter only the essential information. In most practices this includes:
   * The **patient's name.**
   * His **home and work telephone numbers.**
   * A **code** to indicate the service to be performed.

4. Draw an arrow to indicate the length of the appointment.

5. If an appointment is changed, **erase it** — do not cross it out!
   (An appointment book with many visible changes soon becomes a hopeless jumble.)

6. Entries must be made in this order:
   * **First,** write the entry in the appointment book in pencil.
   * **Second,** fill-in the patient's appointment card.
   * **Third,** double check to be certain that the information is complete — and the same in both places.

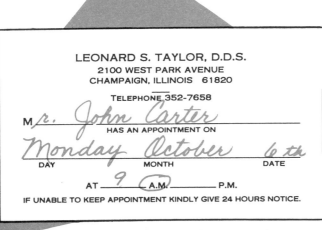

Figure 2-5. A sample appointment card.

THE APPOINTMENT CARD

When an appointment is made for a patient who is in the office, an appointment card is completed and given to the patient. The information on the card also must be complete, legible and accurate (Fig 2-5).

When giving the card to the patient, repeat the time and date of the appointment (Fig 2-6). For example, "*Mrs. Williamson, we've reserved time for you on Monday, January the 21st at 3:30 in the afternoon. We'll be looking forward to seeing you then.*"

The doctor may also request that you add this message: "*If for any reason you cannot keep this appointment, please let us know at least 24 hours in advance.*"

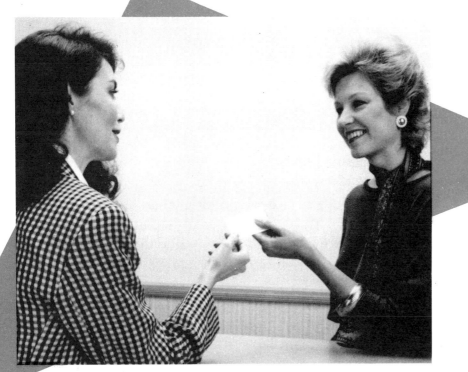

Figure 2-6. As you give the appointment card to the patient, reinforce the appointment day, date and time.

APPOINTMENT SCHEDULING

Effective scheduling is based on knowing **what** is to be done for the patient at the next visit and **how long** this treatment is expected to take.

This information may come from the treatment plan which the dentist has developed for this patient. An alternative is that at the end of the current patient visit, the dentist will specify what is to be done and the length of time needed for the next appointment.

The Scheduling Guide

It is also helpful to have a scheduling guide which is a list of the number of time units the dentist wants reserved for different types of appointments. This should include information on how much time to save for appointments such as:

- ✓ A new patient visit
- ✓ An adult recall patient visit
- ✓ A child recall patient visit
- ✓ A crown preparation
- ✓ Cosmetic dentistry

Many dentists prefer that the most difficult cases be scheduled in the morning or at that time of day when the dentist is feeling his or her best. Throughout the day if possible, a balanced and varied work load should be planned to avoid the negative effects of monotony.

Many dentists, and patients, prefer to plan long appointments so that several procedures can be completed at a single visit. This makes more effective use of the dentist's time and saves the patient from having to make a lot of short visits to the dental office.

As part of the treatment plan the dentist should indicate the number and length of appointments required.

SPECIALIZED SCHEDULING

Just as not all appointments are scheduled for the same length of time, there are other specific needs for certain groups of patients.

Scheduling Emergency Appointments

Buffer time is allowed each day for the treatment of emergencies. The patient experiencing discomfort should be encouraged to come in during buffer time.

However, in a **crisis** situation (such as when a child has fallen and broken a tooth) the patient is usually seen immediately even if this requires the rescheduling of regular patients.

In the event of such an emergency, the situation should be explained to the waiting patients. When they know what has happened, most are very cooperative and understanding about having to wait or change their appointments.

✓	IS THIS AN EMERGENCY?
	How long have you been in pain?
	Does the pain keep you awake at night?
	Is there bleeding?
	Is there swelling?
	Have you broken a tooth?
	Have you lost a filling?
	Do you have a fever?

The Table "*Is This An Emergency?*" contains questions that will help you determine whether or not the caller has an emergency which must be seen immediately or one which can wait until the reserved buffer time.

▶ Scheduling Walk-In Patients

A **walk-in** is a patient who comes to the dental office without having made an appointment. Most frequently the walk-in will be a stranger with a toothache or pain. However, other walk-ins may be potential patients looking for a new dentist.

The manner in which walk-ins are handled depends upon the dentist's policy. Some dentists will not see walk-ins. In this case, the policy is politely explained to the visitor. Sometimes it is helpful to suggest another practice that might be able to help.

Some dentists will try to accommodate the stranger as soon as possible without disrupting regularly scheduled patients. (An emergency patient has the potential of becoming a regular patient within the practice.)

Occasionally the walk-in will be a regular patient who has a dental emergency and decided to come to the office rather than calling for an appointment. In this situation, the dentist usually will make every effort to see the patient as quickly as possible.

▶ Scheduling Work-In Appointments

Brief appointments, which are commonly known as *work-ins,* are used for short procedures such as a denture adjustment, post-operative check or suture removal. Usually these visits can be dove-tailed with the waiting-time that may occur during another appointment.

For example on the schedule shown in Figure 2-7, Mr. Jordan might be worked in for suture removal while Dr. Taylor is waiting for mandibular anesthesia to take effect on George Adams. There is time saved at 11:30 to accommodate an emergency or a walk-in patient.

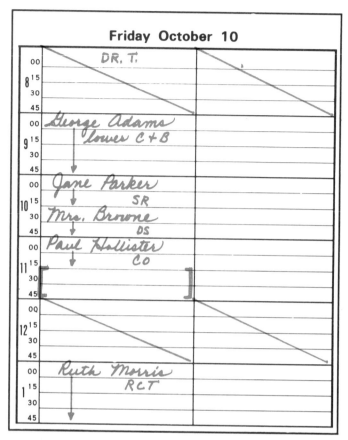

Figure 2-7. Sample schedule with space for work-in and emergency patients.

▶ Scheduling Recall Patients

Recall patients are usually scheduled with the hygienist for x-rays, a prophy (cleaning), a preliminary examination and preventive care instruction. After this, the dentist will see the patient to review the hygienist's findings and to answer questions.

If there is no hygienist, the patient should be scheduled so that an auxiliary has time to take and process the necessary radiographs before the dentist sees the patient.

The time reserved for a recall appointment depends upon the dentist's preference. Most commonly, three units of time are set aside for adults and two for children.

▶ Scheduling Children

Most dentists prefer to see very young children early in the morning (when they are usually feeling their best). This helps to assure that the child will be as cooperative as possible and have a positive experience with his dental treatment. Certainly young children should not be scheduled late in the day when they may be tired and hungry.

School children should be seen (if possible) other than at school times; however, this is not always practical. When school must be missed, a school excuse form should be sent to school with the patient.

A pattern of having school children come in first thing in the morning as they come from home — or immediately after lunch — is more effective than asking that the teacher remember to excuse a child at a certain time.

 ## Scheduling Older Patients

Older patients, who are no longer working, are usually happy to come in during the middle of the day. Some older patients tire easily and prefer not to be scheduled for long appointments.

Scheduling A Series Of Appointments

When scheduling a series of appointments, it is preferable to arrange to have the patient come in at the same time and day of the week throughout the series. This makes it easier for the patients to plan their own schedules and to remember their appointments.

In arranging an appointment series for a service requiring laboratory work (such as dentures or crown and bridge) it is necessary to allow sufficient laboratory working time, including transportation time, between visits.

The Table "*Laboratory Working Time Requirements*" gives examples of the number of laboratory working days, plus a margin for safety, that are required between appointments involving these laboratory services.

The times shown in this Table are hypothetical. It is necessary to generate a list of actual times from the laboratory where cases will be sent.

LABORATORY WORKING TIME REQUIREMENTS					
Full Dentures	**# Days**	**Partial Dentures**	**# Days**	**Inlays, Crowns & Bridges**	**# Days**
Bite blocks, trays	2	Cast partials	7	Direct inlay	2
Set up for try-in	2	Bite blocks	5	Indirect inlay	3
Finish from set up	3	Cast clasps	3	Cast fixed bridge	6
Denture repairs	1	Clasp replacement	4	Gold crown	7
Denture relines	2	Addition to cast partial	5	Porcelain jacket crown	5
Duplicating denture	2	Repairs to partial	1	Acrylic crown	4

CONFIRMATION CALLS

One of the greatest hazards to the orderly flow of services is the patient who fails to keep an appointment, comes at the wrong time, or calls at the last minute to request rescheduling.

A telephone confirmation call the day before the appointment serves as a tactful reminder and helps to prevent many broken appointments.

This approach also makes it possible to catch potential cancellations in time to make maximum use of released time.

When making confirmation calls, try to reach the patient. Even if it requires trying several times, it is best to avoid leaving a message for the patient.

If a scheduled patient visit involves work to be returned by the laboratory, it is a good idea to check that the laboratory work has been completed and returned to the office <u>before</u> making the confirmation call.

Keep the wording of the confirmation call simple and pleasant. For example, "*This is Sue calling from Dr. Taylor's office. I want to confirm that we are looking forward to seeing you tomorrow morning at 10 AM.*"

When the patient has been reached and the appointment confirmed, note this in the appointment book by placing a check mark next to the time of the appointment.

THE DAILY SCHEDULE

Once the appointments have been confirmed, the Daily Schedule Sheets are prepared for the next day (Fig. 2-8). This is done by transferring the following data from the appointment book: the patient's name, appointment time and length, and the treatment planned.

This form serves as a communication control between the business office and the various work centers. A copy should be posted in each operatory, the laboratory, staff lounge and the dentist's private office.

✓ A check mark next to the patient's name indicates that the appointment has been confirmed.

✓ A circle around the time indicates that the appointment has not been confirmed.

✓ Throughout the day as there are changes in the schedule, the daily schedule sheets should be updated.

ADVANCE APPOINTMENT PREPARATION

In preparation for visits of the patients scheduled for the next day, all pertinent patient records should be gathered from the files. These usually include the patient's chart and radiographs and the account ledger card.

These records are usually stored temporarily together in the order in which the patients are to be seen. Charts and radiographs are stored in the filing cabinets where charts are kept. The ledger cards are stored in the ledger card file.

It is also necessary to verify that all laboratory work is ready and has been returned to the office.

```
01-11        DAILY SCHEDULE        Leonard S. Taylor, D.D.S.

TIME      PATIENT NAME          REASON FOR VISIT        ACCOUNT

9:00   ✓Dorothy   Hobson      Crown & Bridge               23

9:15

9:30

9:45

10:00    Lisa      Norman      Restorations                 50

10:15

10:30   ✓Ruth      Green       Endodontic Treatment         31

10:45

11:00   ✓Wallace   Pierce      Denture Service              66

11:15

11:30    Faye      Colson      Toothache                    51

11:45    Lionel    Agnew       Post-Op Check                70

12:00

12:15

12:30

12:45

1:00   ✓Janice    Martin      New Patient                  12

1:15

1:30

1:45   ✓Frances   Newton      Restorations                 61

2:00

2:15
```

Figure 2-8. Computer generated daily schedule sample.

CHANGED APPOINTMENTS

Patients Who Are Late

An office that consistently "runs late" is discourteous to the patients. Therefore, the dentist who is always behind schedule can soon expect that the patients will be late, too. On the other hand, if patients are usually seen on time, they are expected to arrive on time.

There are some people who are chronically late! They are a hazard to an efficient schedule and every effort should be made to "help" them be on time. One technique used, in the hope the habitually late patient will be on time, is state that the appointment is 15 minutes earlier than it is actually scheduled.

Cancelled Appointments

When a patient calls to cancel an appointment, make every effort to get the patient to reschedule the visit as soon as possible.

If the patient cancels and refuses to reschedule, inform the dentist of this fact. Also make an information entry on the patient's chart noting that the patient cancelled the appointment and did not make a new one.

Broken Appointments

When a patient fails to come in for a confirmed appointment, he or she should be contacted as soon as possible to discover the reason and to arrange a new time.

All broken appointments should be noted on the patient's chart because this is contributory negligence on the patient's part. The broken appointment may also be recorded on the account ledger card; however, most dentists do not charge for broken appointments.

Short-Notice Appointments

It is not always easy to fill time made available by a cancellation. One method for doing this is to keep a list of people who can come in on short notice.

These will be patients whose schedules are very flexible, those who can not readily plan ahead for a regular appointment, or those who find anticipating dental work to be worrisome.

Information about these patients should be placed on a file card (Fig. 2-9). You can file these cards in alphabetical order, by categories of priority (emergency, urgent, normal periodic check, etc.), or by the time of day the individual can be free. This file should be kept up-to-date with new names added and outdated ones removed.

When a patient accepts a short-notice appointment, thank him for changing his plans in order to accept this time. You may want to inform the dentist so that he or she too may also acknowledge this.

NAME _Janice Clark_ DATE _1/9/xx_

TELEPHONE NUMBERS   H. _351-4890_   W._____

BEST TIME _mid-morning or early afternoon_

TREATMENT NEEDED _bonding of teeth # 6, 7, 8, 9_

_____

TIME REQUIREMENTS _4 units_

DATE CALLED   RESULTS

_____

_____

_____

Figure 2-9. Short-notice appointment card sample.

Chapter 3

RECORDS MANAGEMENT

LEARNING GOALS

The student will be able to:

▶ State the five basic rules of records protection and the five basic rules for records retrieval.

▶ Name the two major groups of records found in the dental office and list the records that are usually filed together as the "patient chart."

▶ Discuss the importance of patient records and describe the steps to be taken in transferring a record.

▶ Name and describe the five types of filing systems which may be found in a dental office.

▶ Identify the following types of filing equipment and aids: lateral files, drawer files, file guides, out guides, file envelopes and identification labels.

▶ Describe the use of one and two color coding systems and state when each might be used.

▶ Discuss the importance of records retention and the methods used to separate and store active and inactive records.

▶ Define: indexing, caption, unit, alphabetizing, surname, given name, and terms denoting seniority.

▶ Demonstrate arranging names into indexing units and sorting these names into alphabetical order for filing.

OVERVIEW OF RECORDS MANAGEMENT

▶ A filing system is only as good as the findability of everything within the files.

Records management, which is often referred to as **filing**, includes those activities involved in classifying and arranging records so they will be protected and can be retrieved quickly and easily.

The filing system must be organized and maintained so that records are adequately protected and can still be retrieved quickly and easily. The key points here are **protection** and **retrieval!**

▶ Records Protection

The loss of records through fire, flood or other catastrophe could cripple a practice. Therefore, it is important that records be protected at all times. The following are the basic rules for records protection:

1. Original records are not to be taken out of the practice. If this information is needed elsewhere, the document should be photocopied.

2. When not in active use, all records are to be in their proper place in the filing system.

3. At the end of the day, all records are to be returned to the filing system.

4. Before closing the file cabinet, the records are packed tightly together. (This slows fire damage because it does not allow air to circulate between the papers.)

5. At the end of the day, all filing cabinets are closed. (If cabinets are the locking type, they are locked.)

6. Computerized records are protected by making daily and monthly backups. (A **backup** is a copy of the data stored in the system.)

7. The monthly backups are stored away from the office.

▶ Records Retrieval

Each misplaced record creates an unnecessary crisis! Furthermore, searching for lost records is an expensive waste of time.

The most common cause of lost or missing records is "misfiling," that is the failure to return the record to its proper place in the filing system. The following are the basic rules for records retrieval:

1. Having a record in "almost" the right spot is not good enough!

2. Recognize that filing is an important responsibility and never allow yourself to be careless while filing records.

3. Before starting to file, presort the records into approximate alphabetical order.

4. Take the time to get it right the first time. Looking for a misfiled record is time consuming and stressful.

5. Be organized and use adequate filing aids to keep the filing system in top condition.

THE TYPES OF PRACTICE RECORDS

Practice records are divided into two major groups: business records and patient records (Fig. 3-1). These records are maintained in separate filing systems.

▶ Business Records

The business records include all of the information needed to manage the practice and to meet government recordkeeping requirements. These records include:

- All financial data related to patient accounts, including insurance claim information.
- Patient registration forms.
- Bills to be paid.
- Expense records and receipts, including bank statements and cancelled checks.
- Business correspondence and personnel records.
- Records of practice income.
- Annual practice summaries and financial statements.
- Tax records.
- Professional registrations, licenses and insurance policies.

▶ Patient Records

The patient records that are usually stored together and are referred to as the **patient chart** include:

- The **medical and dental history.**
- **Examination and treatment records.** These usually include a tooth chart to record the examination and lines to enter all treatment and other findings.
- **Correspondence** related to the patient's care.
- **Prescriptions and laboratory work orders.**
- **Radiographs,** such as periapical and bite-wing films. Large films, such as extraoral views, are stored in a separate file.

COMPUTERIZED RECORDS MANAGEMENT

The most common application of computerized records management is in accounts receivable bookkeeping. Here, the accounts are identified by numbers, not names.

As with any numerical filing system, this means you must have a way to match the patient's name with his assigned account number. On a computer this is done by **alpha search.** Here is how it works:

- ✓ Simply type the first several letters of the patient's last name.
- ✓ The system will display a list of the first and last names (and account numbers) of all patients with similar last names.
- ✓ Select the correct name, type the account number and proceed with the function.

40

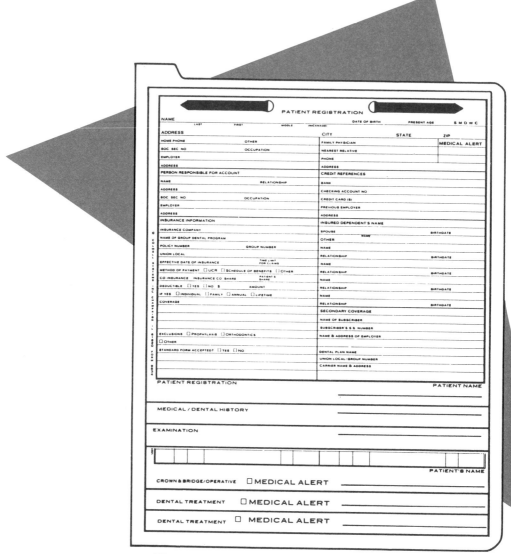

Figure 3-1. A fully integrated patient chart in a manila file folder with a fastener added.

There are also software programs available that will manage all of the patient's clinical records. In dentistry, it is difficult for a computerized record to completely replace a patient chart because it is still necessary to maintain a file for the patient's radiographs.

THE IMPORTANCE OF PATIENT RECORDS

 Legal Documents

 Patient records are important legal documents.

Patient records are important legal documents which must be preserved. Therefore, each patient's chart must be maintained in good order so that all parts of the record are clear and well organized.

Financial records, such as ledger cards and insurance claims, are <u>not</u> part of the patient's clinical record. They should be stored with business records — not as part of the patient's chart.

▶ Maintaining Confidentiality

Patient records contain confidential information which must be protected. Records should be managed so that confidential information is not left lying around where it might be seen by another patient or unauthorized person.

▶ The Ownership Of Patient Records

Occasionally the question arises as to *"Who owns the patient's chart?"* One way of looking at this is that the dentist owns the actual chart and the patient owns the information contained within the chart.

Under law, the patient must be allowed reasonable access to this data. For example, on request, the patient should be allowed to see the contents of his chart.

However, no one other than practice employees may review this information regarding the patient's treatment without the patient's consent.

▶ The Transfer Of Patient Records

Because patient charts are important legal documents, the dentist may refuse to allow the original chart to leave the office except under a court order.

When it is necessary to transfer records, a photocopy of the chart may be sent in place of the original. When this is done, a note is made on the original chart as to the date and where the copy was sent.

Also, original radiographs are not allowed to leave the practice. Instead, duplicates are made of the radiographs and the duplicate is sent with the records.

An alternative to copying the entire record, is to send a summary of the past two or three years of the patient's record. If a summary is created, a copy of this should be filed with the patient's original records.

✓ The doctor may charge a small fee to cover the copying and clerical expenses involved in transferring the record.

✓ The doctor <u>may not</u> refuse to release the patient's records just because the bill has not been paid.

However, before any information can be transferred, the patient is asked to sign a written **Release of Information** form which grants the doctor permission to give out this information.

TYPES OF FILING SYSTEMS

Not all records for the practice are stored in a single filing system. Instead, several different types of specialized filing systems are maintained to accommodate different records needs.

▶ Subject Filing

In subject filing, all files are labeled according to the subject of their contents. These folders are then filed alphabetically. Subject filing is commonly used for business records.

Chronological Filing

Chronological filing organizes information according to time spans such as months and days (Fig. 3-2). Chronological files are frequently used for the recall system.

This type of system may also be used as a **tickler** or **come-up file** to remind you of important tasks that are performed on a periodic basis.

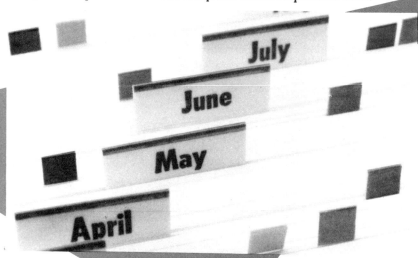

Figure 3-2. A chronological file is frequently used for the recall system.

Filing Radiographs

It may be necessary to store radiographs not in the patient chart, but as a separate file. In this case, they are usually organized and filed under the same type of system that is used to file patient records. This would be alphabetical or numerical filing. To assure greater accuracy, these files should also be clearly labeled and color coded.

Alphabetical Filing

Alphabetical filing is commonly used for records such as patient charts and ledger cards.

With alphabetical filing, all items are filed in strict alphabetical order following the rules of indexing which are discussed at the end of this chapter.

Numerical Filing

▶ People have names, not numbers.

In numerical filing each chart or document is assigned a number. Computerized systems usually access records by account number. This is a form of numerical filing.

Straight numerical filing is the most commonly used form of numerical filing. It has all items filed in 1-2-3 order so that number 125 would follow 124 and precede 126.

Generally, numerical filing is used for patient records only in practices with more than 20,000 active patient charts.

An exception to this rule is when patient records are maintained on the computer. In computerized systems, the record is assigned a number and is retrieved by accessing that number.

People have names — not numbers. Therefore, whenever numerical filing is used, it is necessary to maintain a cross-reference file to find the number assigned to that patient record.

▶ Cross-Reference Filing

A cross-reference filing is an alphabetical listing which makes it possible to locate materials that have been filed numerically. For ease of access, these listings are usually organized as a rotary file.

FILING AIDS AND EQUIPMENT

▶ Drawer Files

Drawer files are also known as **vertical files.** These drawers provide good protection for their contents.

This type of file may be used for patient records; however, drawer files are most often used to store practice business records (Fig. 3-3).

▶ Lateral Files

Lateral files are also know as **open shelf filing.** This type of file, which provides easy access and is particularly well adapted to color coding, is commonly used for patient records (Fig. 3- 4).

▶ File Guides

File guides are used to better organize the files by identifying major groups of files. There are two types of file guides:

✓ **Primary guides** that are used for the main subject, letter of the alphabet or the numerical headings.
✓ **Auxiliary guides** that establish subdivisions within these primary categories.

The greater the number of guides, the more accurate and rapid the filing and retrieving will be. Depending upon the thickness of the files, having a guide for every ten to twenty folders or envelopes usually works well.

▶ Out Guides

Out guides serve as bookmarks for the filing system. As such they make refiling faster and facilitate spotting the "home" of charts to be returned to the file (Fig. 3-5).

These guides should be brightly colored and slightly larger than the other file folders so that they will be easier to see.

An out guide must always be placed where a chart is removed from the file. It is easier to do this if the out guides are kept in a convenient place where they are easy to reach. This might be in the front of each file drawer or at the end of each file shelf.

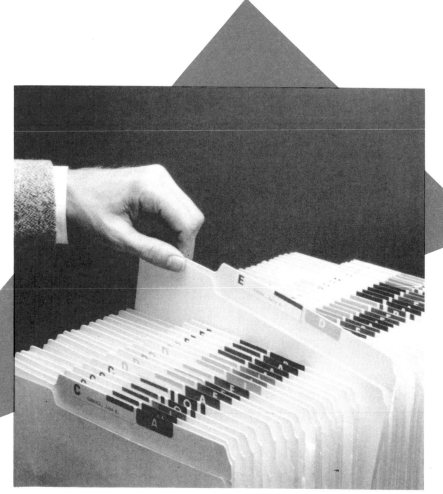

Figure 3-3. Drawer files are used most frequently for business records.

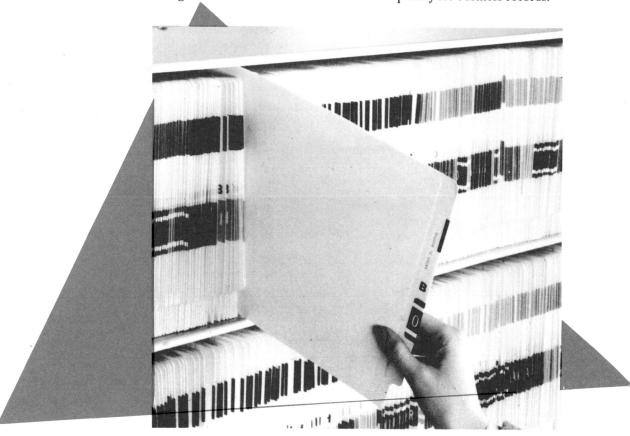

Figure 3-4. Lateral files and color coding make an excellent combination for organizing and managing patient charts.

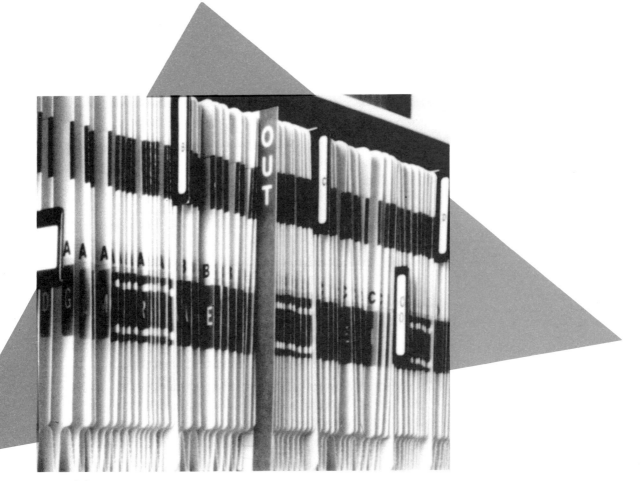

Figure 3-5. Out guides serve as bookmarks for the filing system.

File Envelopes

File envelopes, which are closed on three sides, are a light-weight means of storing and protecting patient records.

File envelopes have the advantage that they are an effective means of holding all records together. This is desirable if there are small radiographs or notes in the chart.

Unfortunately, it is usually necessary to empty all of the contents of the envelope in order to access any part of the record.

File Folders

Manila file folders are more durable and have added strength to protect patient records.

A fastener, dividers or plastic pocket may be added to the inside of the folder to help organize papers and to hold them securely in place.

The File Label

Each file folder or envelope must be clearly marked with a typewritten identification label.

- With **drawer filing,** identification information is placed across the top of the file folder.
- With **shelf filing,** identification information is placed down the side of the file folder.

The name on the label must be complete so that it is possible to select the correct chart without having to sort through the contents.

The name should be arranged on the label in the same sequence that is used for alphabetical indexing. For example, the label for *John David Jones, Jr.,* would be typed as shown below:

> *JONES, JOHN DAVID JR.*

▶ Ageing Tabs

Ageing tabs, which are also known as **purge tabs,** are a color coding system that speeds sorting active and inactive charts (Fig. 3-6). The tab for each year is color coded and shows the two last digits of that year.

Here is how they work. The first time Mr. Jones visited in 1991, a red *"91"* tab is placed in his chart. Each time he returns in 1991, nothing more is done with this. On his first visit in 1992, a green *"92"* tab is placed over the 1991 label. If Mr. Jones does not return in 1992, nothing is changed.

Then, when it is time to sort active/inactive charts, it is easy to simply pick out the inactive records by spotting the appropriately colored tab.

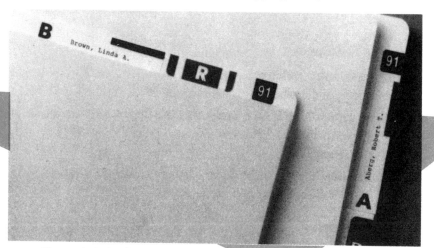

Figure 3-6. Ageing tabs speed sorting active and inactive charts.

COLOR CODING FILES

Color coding speeds filing and reduces the number of "lost charts" due to misfiling. It may be used effectively with either alphabetical or numerical filing systems.

The color coding labels on the charts form a pattern that makes a misfiled chart easy to spot.

Color coding labels come in a mixture of solid colors and stripes to create 26 different combinations. Each label also has the appropriate letter printed on it.

Records may be color coded using either one, two or three colors. The number of colors used is determined by the number of records to be actively managed in the practice.

An "average" figure is about four to six records per inch; however, this will vary greatly from one practice to another.

To estimate how many patient records are in the files, count the number of records in twelve inches and multiply this by the total amount of file space in use.

 ## Single Color Coding

A single color label, or a colored file envelope, is coded for the first letter of the patient's last name (Fig. 3-7).

Since colored file envelopes only come in ten colors, each color must be repeated in order to accommodate the entire alphabet.

Single color coding works well on business records and for patient charts in a small practice with up to 2,000 active files.

However, since two color coding is so much more efficient, many small practices use it to save time in filing and in looking for lost charts!

 ## Two Color Coding

Two color coding is used very effectively in practices with 2,000 to 10,000 active records. The majority of practices fall into this range.

Two color labels are coded using the first two letters of the patient's last name (Figs. 3-8 through 3-10). For example, the chart for *John David Jones, Jr.,* would be tagged with a red "J" label and a blue "O" label.

Three Color Coding

Three color labels are used to code <u>either</u> for the first two letters of the patient's last name and the first letter of the patient's first name, <u>or</u> to code the first three letters of the patient's last name (Fig. 3-11).

Three color coding is recommended for practices with between 10,000 and 20,000 active records. However, this range is considered to be a transition area.

Some practices, near the low end of the range, stay with two color coding and make every effort to control the size of their active files.

Practices, in the middle of the range, use three color coding. Practices near the high end, and anticipating further growth, go to a numerical filing system combined with color coding.

USING COLOR CODED NAME LABELS

Step 1

Insert label strip into the typewriter with alphabetical character corresponding to first letter of the surname to the left.

Type surname, given name and middle initial. This patient's name is *AMBER, ROBERT T.*

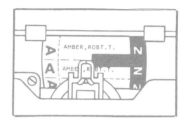

Step 2

Remove label from backing sheet leaving the undesired alphabetical character (located on the right side of the label) on the backing sheet. The label now should measure 3-2/8" x 1-1/4".

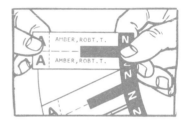

Step 3

Attach label to folder and then add the second label to code the second letter of the last name.

The illustration shows proper positioning of the label for either top tab or side tab file folders.

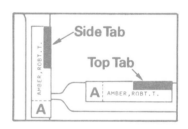

Step 4

Reversing the name labels in the typewriter changes the color coding. For example, to color code the name *NELSON, JOHN R.,* place the label in the typewriter with the "N" to the left. This makes it possible to code all 26 letters of the alphabet with only 13 different name labels.

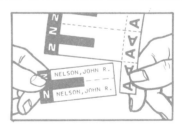

Figure 3-7. The steps in applying color coded name labels.

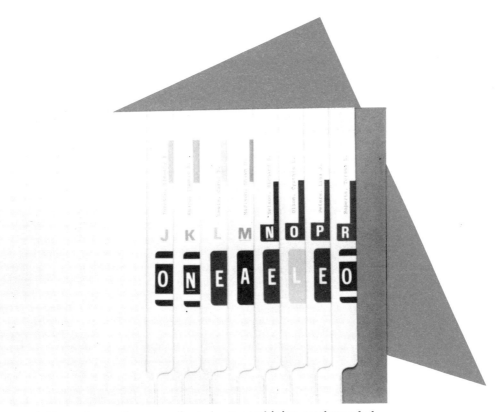

Figure 3-8. Two color coding on patient charts combining a color coded name label with a second color tag.

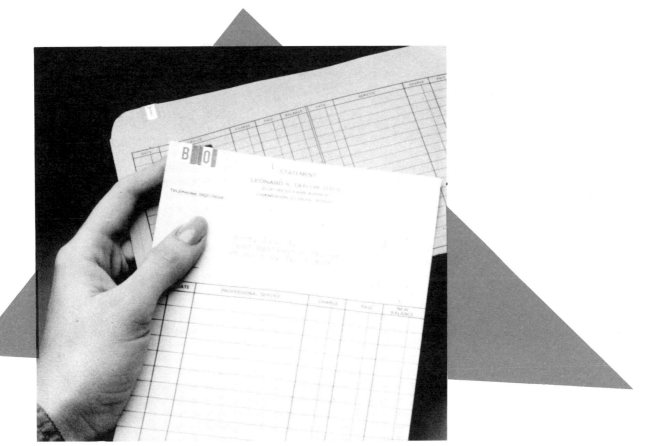

Figure 3-9. Two color coding on a patient ledger card and on a colored file envelope

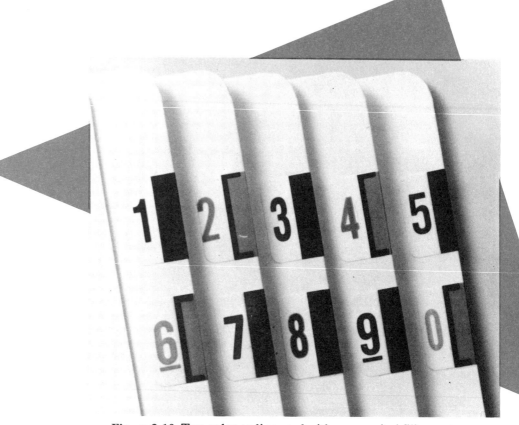

Figure 3-10. Two color coding used with a numerical filing system.

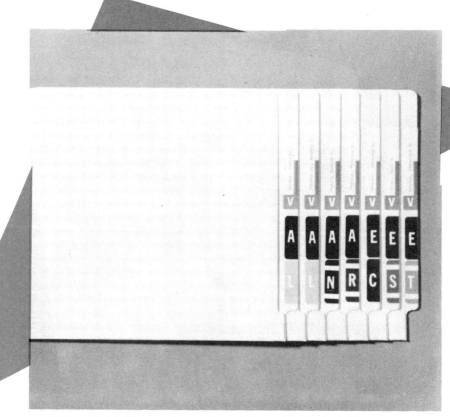

Figure 3-11. Three color coding with an alphabetical filing system.

RECORDS RETENTION

The retention schedule for practice business records differs according to the type of records. For example, different guidelines apply as to how long paid ledger cards and unpaid ledger cards, or Medicare and Medicaid remittance information must be kept.

However, the guidelines for clinical patient records are much clearer. Patient charts are important legal documents which are classified as permanent records. This means that they should not be discarded.

With both types of records, there is one basic rule. Never discard any records without the doctor's permission. Also, keep all records in an orderly manner so that they may be retrieved as necessary.

Controlling file size is an important part of records management. Each extra record that must be sorted through daily slows filing and retrieving records and increases the possibility for error. Also, records suffer from the wear and tear of constant handling.

Rather than simply letting the files grow, or switching to a more complex filing system, it is desirable to control file size by periodically removing inactive records.

▶ Never discard any record without the doctor's permission!

▶ Active Files

Active files are stored in the area that is easiest to reach for day-to-day use. These are the charts for patients who are being seen regularly, or who have been seen recently.

- If the file shelves extend from floor to ceiling, the middle shelves, which are the most convenient to use, are used to store the active files.
- If file space in the business office is very limited, all of this space is considered to be active.

▶ Inactive Files

Inactive files are the records of patients who have not been seen in the past three years. These charts are stored in space that is still accessible, but not quite as convenient as the active file area.

- In the floor to ceiling file, the top shelves are considered to be inactive or secondary file space.
- If all of the business office files are classified as being active, the inactive files may be maintained in a storage room or basement.
- These records must be kept dry and safe, and in good order so that they can be retrieved as necessary.

▶ Storage Files

A storage file is maintained in an out-of-the-way location and is used for storing charts of patients who have died or are no longer with the practice.

- These records still must be properly protected and kept in an organized manner so that a file can be retrieved if necessary.

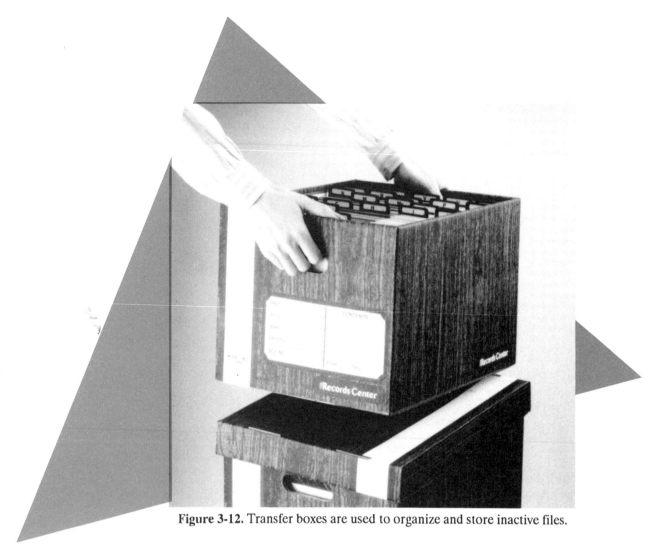

Figure 3-12. Transfer boxes are used to organize and store inactive files.

- Records in this category are often stored in cardboard transfer boxes (Fig. 3-12).
- Each box must be clearly labeled as to the contents.

▶ Sorting Active And Inactive Files

The frequency with which active and inactive files are sorted depends upon the doctor's preference, the type of practice, and the amount of active file space that is available.

Generally, inactive files are removed from the active file once a year. As previously described, the use of ageing tabs greatly speeds and simplifies this process.

When charts are transferred from the active to the inactive files, they must be added to these files in alphabetical order. Then, when searching the inactive files, it should be necessary to look only in one place to find the record.

When transferring records to the inactive file, radiographs may be removed from their mount and placed in an envelope which is clearly labeled with the patient's name and the date the films were taken.

When transferring records from the inactive file into storage, they are often stored by year. When doing this, it is necessary to create an inventory for each box, which lists the full name shown on each patient chart in that box.

RULES FOR INDEXING
FOR ALPHABETICAL FILING

The following are the rules for indexing which must be followed when preparing records for alphabetical filing. (**Indexing** is the process of determining the order in which the units of a name are to be considered.)

▶ Division Into Units

Names to be filed alphabetically are organized into indexing units. The units are filed in strict alphabetical order.

These indexing units for alphabetical filing are based on the surname, first name, middle name and terms denoting seniority.

- **UNIT I — The surname.** This is the family name (last name) of an individual.
- **UNIT II — The given name.** This is the individual's first name.
- **UNIT III — The middle name.** This may be a given name, an initial, or a woman's maiden name.
- **UNIT IV — Terms denoting seniority.** These include "Junior," "Senior", and "III."

The chart below shows how the name *John David Jones, Jr.,* would be arranged into indexing units.

I	II	III	IV
Jones	*John*	*David*	*Junior*
surname	first name	middle name	seniority term

▶ Nothing Comes Before Something

A surname alone precedes the same surname with a first name or initial. A surname with a first initial only precedes the same surname with a complete first name beginning with the same letter as the initial.

I	II	III	IV
Black			
Black	*R.*		
Black	*Robert*		
Black	*Robert*	*W.*	
Black	*Robert*	*William*	
Black	*Robert*	*William*	*Jr.*

▶ **Prefixes**

A prefix is part of a surname and the entire last name is considered as a single indexing unit. Last names are arranged in strict alphabetical order before first names or middle initials are taken into consideration.

I	II	III	IV
MacNeal	Arthur	A.	
MacNeil	Angus	G.	
McLain	Andrew	Robert	
McLean	Alice	F.	

▶ **Abbreviated Prefixes**

An abbreviation, such as the "St." in St. John, is indexed as if it were spelled out Saint John. However, it is still considered as part of the first indexing unit with the balance of the surname.

I	II	III	IV
St. John	Francis	Lee	Jr.

The following table shows how the name St. John (Saint John) would be handled in an alphabetical file.

I	II	III	IV
Sabin	Joseph	Walter	III
St. John	Francis	Lee	Jr.
Samsone	Agnes	G.	(Mrs.)

▶ **Hyphenated Names**

Hyphenated names are indexed as one unit and are filed in strict alphabetical order.

I	II	III	IV
Smith-Jay	Henry	David	Sr.

The following table shows how the name Smith-Jay would be handled in an alphabetical file.

I	II	III	IV
Smith	Hazel		
Smith-Jay	Henry	David	Sr.
Smythe	Hubert	W.	Jr.

Titles And Degrees

Titles and degrees are not indexing units unless they differentiate between two names that are otherwise exactly the same. They may be added in parentheses for information only.

I	II	III	IV
LaRue	Laura	T.	(Ph.D.)
Lawson	Clarence	W.	
Lawson	Clarence	W.	(M.D.)

Terms Denoting Seniority

Terms such as "Junior" and "Senior" that denote seniority are indexing units and are handled in straight alphabetical order.

A roman numeral is alphabetized as if it were spelled out. For example, III is indexed as "third."

I	II	III	IV
Parker	Stephen	F.	Junior
Parker	Stephen	F.	Senior
Parker	Stephen	F.	III

The Names Of Married Women

A woman's legal name is the one used for indexing. This usually consists of her husband's surname; her given name; her middle name, initial or maiden name. "Mrs." and her husband's first name may be enclosed in parentheses for information purposes; however, they do not affect filing.

The name of a woman who has not taken her husband's last name is indexed as if she were single; however, the name of her husband may be entered for information only.

I	II	III	IV
Harris	Barbara	Jane	(Mrs. T. Nelson)
Jones	Mary	Black	(Mrs. John D.)

Chapter

DENTAL CHARTING AND TERMINOLOGY

LEARNING GOALS

The student will be able to:

▶ Describe the role of an endodontist, oral surgeon, orthodontist, pediatric dentist, periodontist and prosthodontist.

▶ Define or identify: dentition, edentulous, quadrants, interproximal, and the type of teeth.

▶ Identify the letter abbreviations used to describe the surfaces of the teeth.

▶ Describe Black's five classifications of cavities.

▶ Identify anatomical and geometric tooth diagrams.

▶ State how to correct a charting error

▶ Demonstrate using the Universal Numbering System to identify the permanent and primary teeth

▶ Demonstrate recording a dental examination and dental treatment using the appropriate charting symbols and abbreviations.

OVERVIEW OF DENTAL CHARTING AND TERMINOLOGY

All business office employees need to understand basic dental terminology. They must also be able to read the charting entries. This information is used in planning appointments, accounts receivable bookkeeping, completing insurance claims and answering questions (Fig. 4-1).

COMPUTERIZED DENTAL CHARTING

A computer may be used to record the dental examination. As the findings are dictated by the dentist, the assistant keys this information into the system. Here, as with manual charting, it is essential that the data be entered into the system accurately.

The system then prints a diagrammatic representation of the results (similar to the diagram found on a dental chart). This print-out becomes part of the patient's chart.

Another option is a computerized periodontal probe which is used to accurately measure and record the depth of periodontal pockets. The printed report becomes part of the patient's chart.

BASIC DENTAL TERMINOLOGY

► The Dental Specialties

A general practitioner may refer patients to these dental specialists:

- An **endodontist** treats diseases and injuries of the dental pulp. This treatment is called *endodontics* or *root canal therapy.*
- An **oral surgeon** specializes in the surgical treatment of diseases, injuries, and defects involving the teeth and the hard and soft tissues of the oral and maxillofacial regions.

  Patients are commonly referred to an oral surgeon for difficult extractions such as the removal of an impacted third molar.
- An **orthodontist** is a specialist in the correction of all forms of malocclusion.

  Malocclusion is when the teeth are not positioned in the proper relationship to each other.
- A **pediatric dentist** usually treats children from birth through adolescence. Most children are treated by the general practitioner.
- A **periodontist** is concerned with the diagnosis and treatment of disease of the gingival tissues (gums and bone) which surround and support the teeth.
- A **prosthodontist** specializes in the replacement of missing teeth. This specialty is divided into fixed and removable prosthetics.

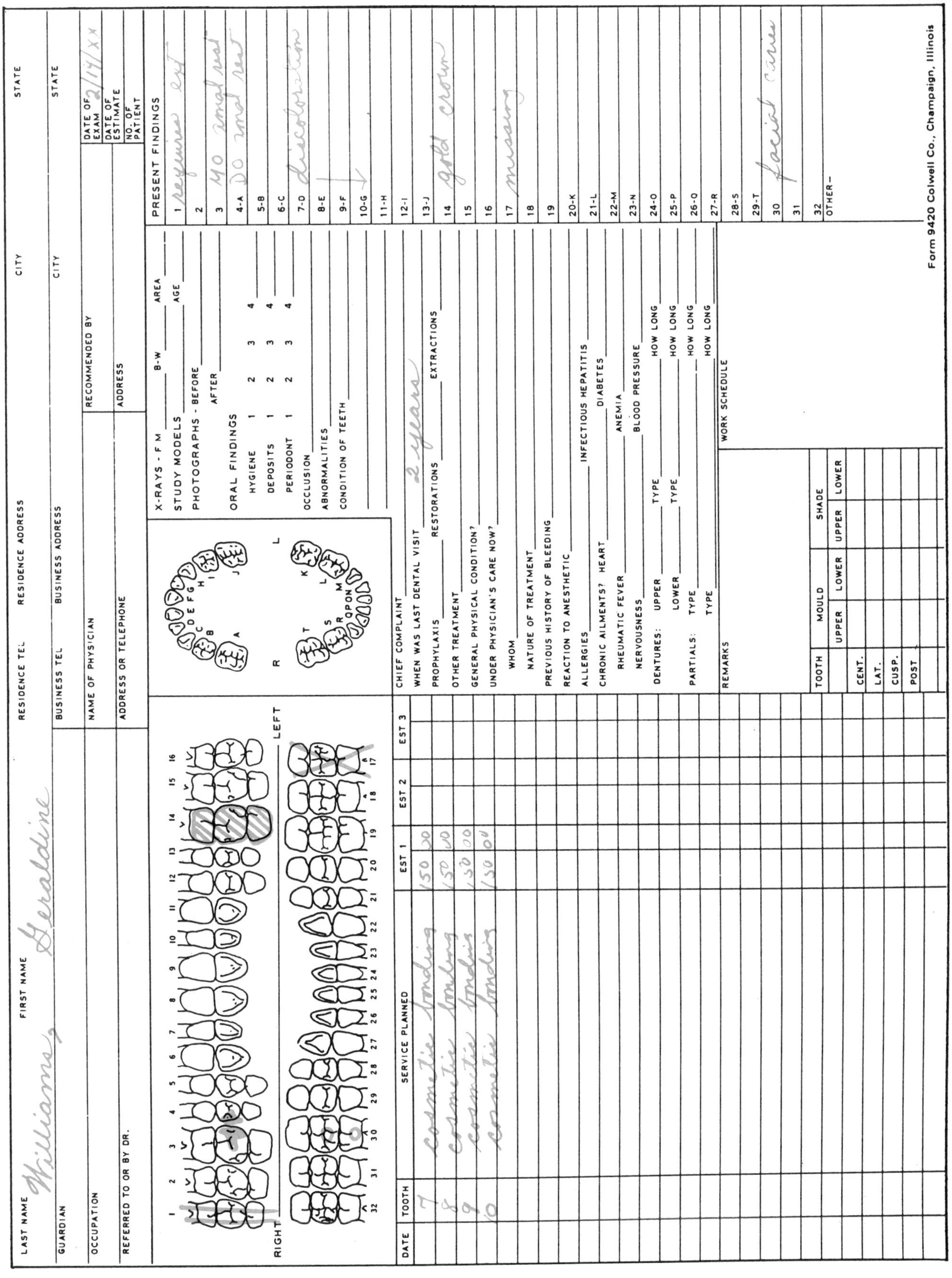

Figure 4-1. Letter size patient chart (front only).

Fixed prosthetics is commonly referred to as **crown and bridge.** Here the missing teeth are replaced with an appliance that is cemented in place and cannot be removed by the patient.

A **bridge** is an appliance which replaces one or two missing teeth. It is described by the number of units involved:

✓ A **pontic** is a unit which replaces a missing tooth.
✓ An **abutment** is a natural tooth which holds the pontic in place. There is usually an abutment at both ends of the bridge.

A **crown** is a restoration that completely covers the crown of the tooth. Crowns are commonly placed on the abutment teeth; however, a crown may also be used to cover an individual tooth that is not part of a bridge.

Removable Prosthetics

Removable prosthetics is the replacement of missing teeth with an appliance that can be placed and removed by the patient.

✓ When all of the teeth in an arch are missing, a **full denture** is placed.
✓ When some teeth in an arch are missing and some are still remaining, a **partial denture** may be placed.

The Jaws

The term **dentition** means the natural teeth in the dental arch. The term **edentulous** means without teeth, and refers to having lost all of the natural teeth.

The **primary dentition,** commonly known as the *baby teeth*, consists of 20 teeth. The **permanent dentition** consists of 32 teeth which are designed to last a lifetime.

The upper jaw is the **maxillary arch.** The lower jaw is the **mandibular arch.** Each arch is divided by an imaginary line into **quadrants. A quadrant** is one of four sections (Fig 4-2). The quadrants of the mouth are the:

● Maxillary right quadrant.
● Maxillary left quadrant.
● Mandibular right quadrant.
● Mandibular left quadrant.

The Types Of Teeth

The Anterior Teeth

The anterior teeth are the front teeth that can be seen when you smile. These include the **central incisors, lateral incisors** and the **cuspids.**

Anterior teeth have **incisal edges** for cutting and tearing food. There is one of each of these types of teeth in each quadrant of the primary and permanent dentition.

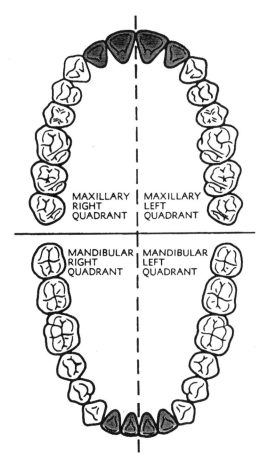

Figure 4-2. Diagram showing division into quadrants.
(The anterior teeth are shaded. The posterior teeth are not shaded.)

The Posterior Teeth

The posterior teeth are the back teeth that are used for chewing. These include the **premolars** and the **molars.**

Posterior teeth have **occlusal surfaces** for chewing and grinding food. There are two premolars and three molars in each quadrant of the permanent dentition. There are two molars, but no premolars, in each quadrant of the primary dentition.

▶ The Tooth Surfaces

The Table "*Abbreviations Used To Identify Tooth Surfaces*" gives the names of the tooth surfaces and the abbreviations which are often used to describe and record dental conditions and treatment.

The term **interproximal** means between the teeth. The mesial and distal surfaces are the interproximal surfaces of each tooth.

When more than one surface is involved in the description, the letters are combined. For example, MO for the mesial and occlusal surfaces. MOD for mesial, occlusal and distal surfaces.

ABBREVIATIONS USED TO IDENTIFY TOOTH SURFACES		
D	**Distal:** The interproximal tooth surface that is <u>away from</u> the midline.
F	**Facial:** The tooth surface that is nearest the cheek or lips.
I	**Incisal:** The cutting edge of an anterior tooth.
L	**Lingual:** The tooth surface that is nearest the tongue.
M	**Mesial:** The interproximal tooth surface that is <u>toward</u> the midline.
O	**Occlusal:** The chewing surface of a posterior tooth.

THE UNIVERSAL NUMBERING SYSTEM

The Universal Numbering System was adopted in 1968 by the American Dental Association to assure accuracy in identification and description of the teeth, and to increase the speed of dictation and transcription of information.

► The Permanent Dentition

As shown in the Table "*The Universal Numbering System For The Permanent Teeth,*" with this system the permanent teeth are numbered from one to thirty-two starting with #1, the maxillary right third molar, continuing around to #16, the maxillary left third molar, then dropping to #17, the mandibular left third molar and working around to #32 the mandibular right third molar.

THE UNIVERSAL NUMBERING SYSTEM FOR THE PERMANENT TEETH			
#	**Maxillary Teeth**	#	**Mandibular Teeth**
1	Maxillary right third molar	17	Mandibular left third molar
2	Maxillary right second molar	18	Mandibular left second molar
3	Maxillary right first molar	19	Mandibular left first molar
4	Maxillary right second premolar	20	Mandibular left second premolar
5	Maxillary right first premolar	21	Mandibular left first premolar
6	Maxillary right cuspid	22	Mandibular left cuspid
7	Maxillary right lateral incisor	23	Mandibular left lateral incisor
8	Maxillary right central incisor	24	Mandibular left central incisor
9	Maxillary left central incisor	25	Mandibular right central incisor
10	Maxillary left lateral incisor	26	Mandibular right lateral incisor
11	Maxillary left cuspid	27	Mandibular right cuspid
12	Maxillary left first premolar	28	Mandibular right first premolar
13	Maxillary left second premolar	29	Mandibular right second premolar
14	Maxillary left first molar	30	Mandibular right first molar
15	Maxillary left second molar	31	Mandibular right second molar
16	Maxillary left third molar	32	Mandibular right third molar

The Primary Dentition

As shown in the Table, "*The Universal Numbering System For The Primary Teeth,*" the primary teeth are lettered from A to T starting with **A**, the maxillary right second molar continuing around to **J** the maxillary second molar, then dropping to **K**, the mandibular left second molar and working around to **T** the mandibular right second molar.

CAVITY CLASSIFICATIONS

The dentist uses Black's system of cavity classification as a shorthand way of describing the types and locations of cavities and restorations.

Class I: Pit And Fissure Cavities

Class I cavities occur primarily in the pits and fissures (natural grooves and indentations) on the occlusal surfaces of the posterior teeth.

Class II: Posterior Interproximal Cavities

Class II cavities occur in the occlusal and interproximal surfaces of premolars and molars. These cavities are named for the surfaces involved. For example, a DO involves the distal and occlusal surfaces.

Class III: Anterior Interproximal Cavities

Class III cavities occur in the interproximal (mesial and distal) surfaces of anterior teeth.

Class IV: Anterior Interproximal Cavities Involving The Incisal Angle

Class IV cavities occur in the interproximal surfaces of incisors and cuspids and involve the incisal angle of that tooth. For example, the corner of an anterior tooth is involved and would be described as either a MI (mesial-incisal) or DI (distal-incisal) Class IV.

Class V: Smooth Surface Cavities

Class V cavities occur near the gum line on the facial or lingual surfaces of any tooth. These are also described as *root caries.*

CHARTING THE DENTAL EXAMINATION

The initial examination, and all recall examinations, are recorded on the patient's chart. There are many styles of charts available so that the dentist may select the type that best suits his or her practice (Figs. 4-1 and 4-3).

When a preprinted chart does not meet the dentist's needs, it is possible to have a special chart designed and printed through a custom printing service.

THE UNIVERSAL NUMBERING SYSTEM FOR THE PRIMARY TEETH			
#	**Maxillary Teeth**	#	**Mandibular Teeth**
A	Maxillary right second molar	K	Mandibular left second molar
B	Maxillary right first molar	L	Mandibular left first molar
C	Maxillary right cuspid	M	Mandibular left cuspid
D	Maxillary right lateral incisor	N	Mandibular left lateral incisor
E	Maxillary right central incisor	O	Mandibular left central incisor
F	Maxillary left central incisor	P	Mandibular right central incisor
G	Maxillary left lateral incisor	Q	Mandibular right lateral incisor
H	Maxillary left cuspid	R	Mandibular right cuspid
I	Maxillary left first molar	S	Mandibular right first molar
J	Maxillary left second molar	T	Mandibular right second molar

▶ Tooth Diagrams

Dental charts include a diagram of the teeth which is used to record examination findings.

- ✓ **Geometric diagrams** use circles to indicate the teeth and their surfaces (Fig. 4-4).
- ✓ **Anatomical diagrams** are a two-dimensional representation of the actual structures and surfaces of the teeth. Some include only the crowns of the teeth (Figs. 4-5 and 4-6). Others also show the root surfaces.
- ✓ Periodontal charts have an anatomical diagram plus space to record pocket depths and lines to indicate the level of gingival recession and bone loss (Fig. 4-7).

▶ Left And Right Quadrants

The teeth in these diagrams are arranged as if you were looking at them from a position on the patient's tongue. This puts:

- ✓ The **right quadrants** are on the **left side** of the page.
- ✓ The **left quadrants** are on the **right side** of the page.

▶ Charting Symbols

Each dentist uses symbols to record clinical data on the charting diagram. The symbols used are based on the dentist's personal preference. Some of the more commonly used symbols are shown in Figure 4-8; however, these can be confusing. For example, as shown here, two parallel lines mean that the tooth is to be extracted. In other systems, two parallel lines mean that the tooth is missing.

When working with charting symbols, always double check that you understand the meaning of the symbols being used in this practice.

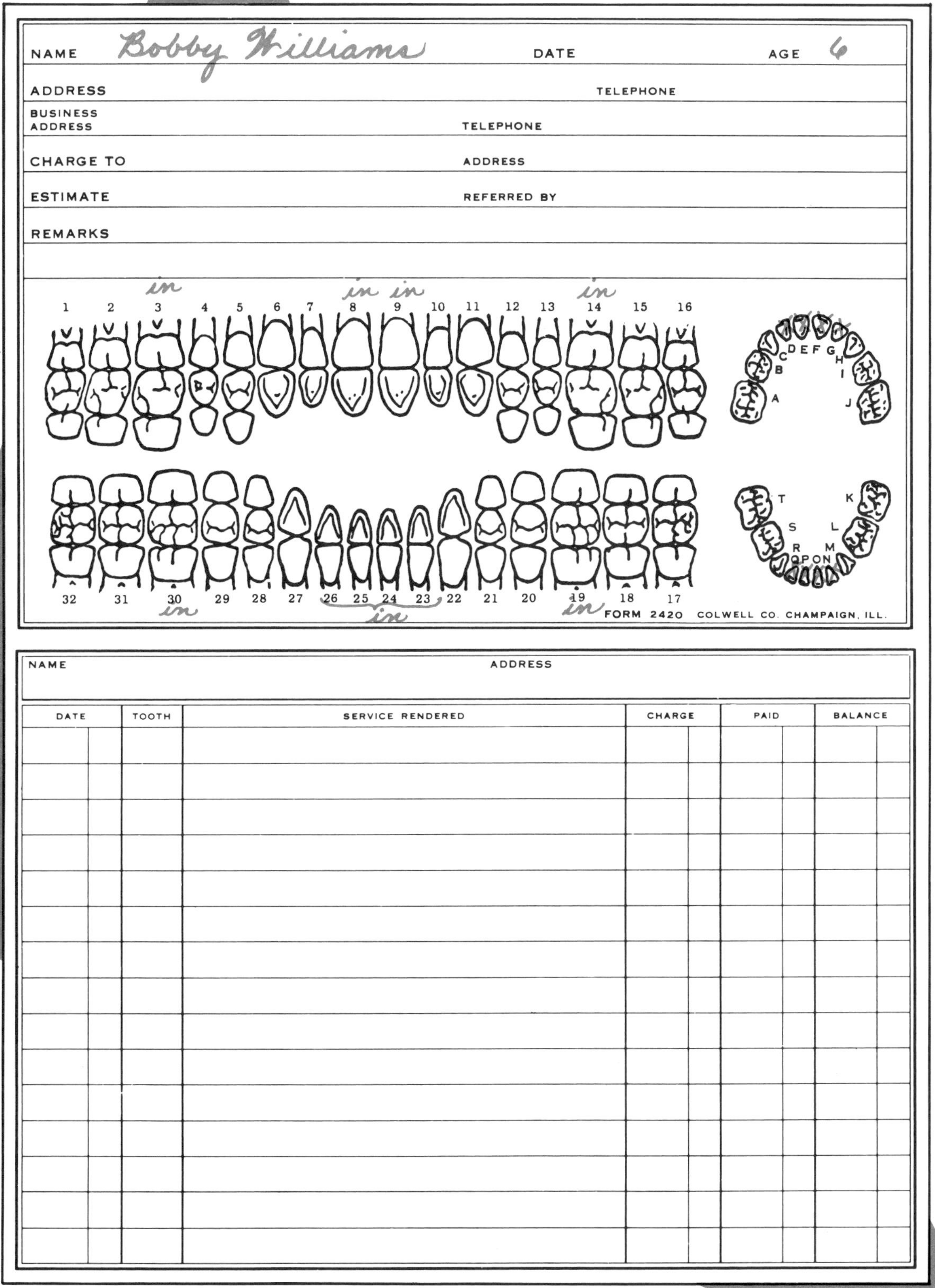
NAME Bobby Williams DATE AGE 6

ADDRESS TELEPHONE

BUSINESS ADDRESS TELEPHONE

CHARGE TO ADDRESS

ESTIMATE REFERRED BY

REMARKS

FORM 2420 COLWELL CO. CHAMPAIGN, ILL.

NAME ADDRESS

DATE	TOOTH	SERVICE RENDERED	CHARGE	PAID	BALANCE

Figure 4-3. Folder style patient chart.

66

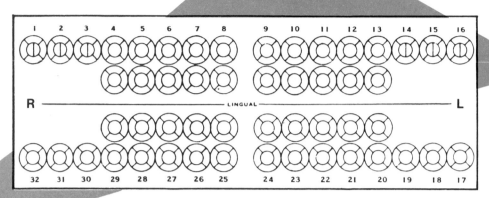

Figure 4-4. A geometric tooth diagram showing both the primary and permanent teeth.

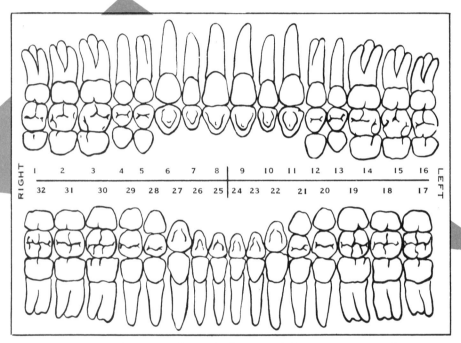

Figure 4-5. An anatomic tooth diagram of the permanent teeth.

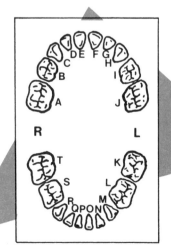

Figure 4-6. A tooth diagram of the primary teeth (occlusal view).

67

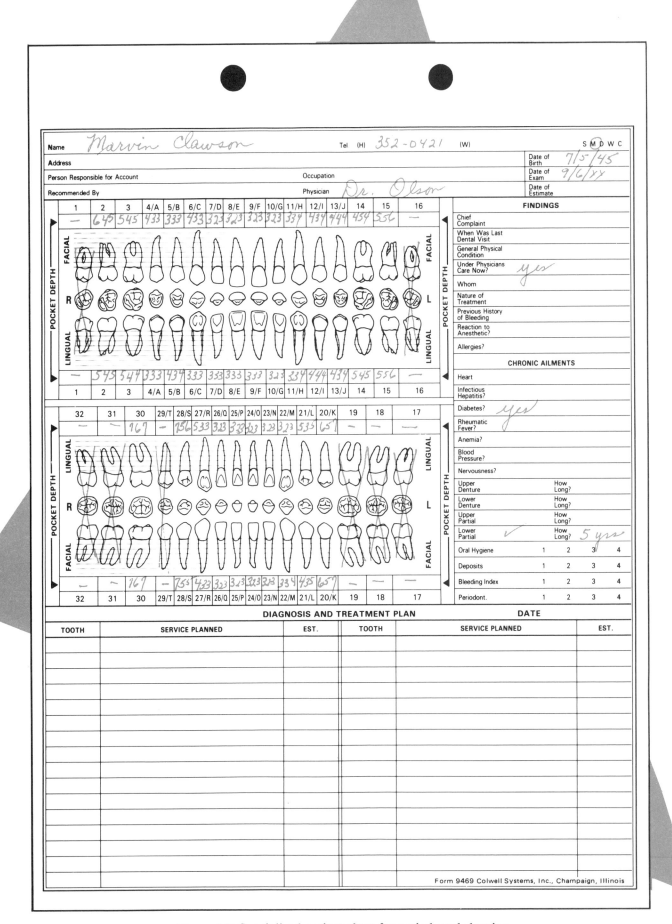

Figure 4-7. Specialized patient chart for periodontal charting.

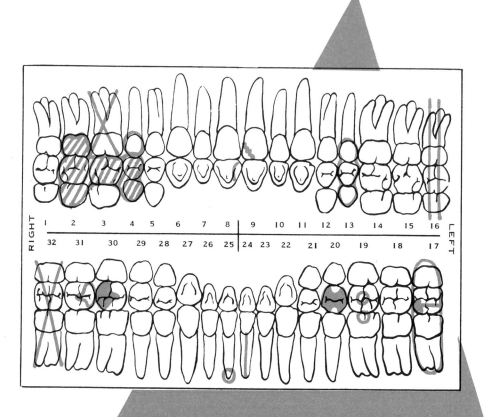

#	CONDITION
2	**Full crown, abutment for bridge.** Cross-hatching indicates a gold restoration.
3	**Missing,** replaced with a pontic. The missing tooth is indicated with an X. The gold pontic is shown with cross-hatching.
4	**Veneer crown, abutment for bridge.** This is a full crown with the facial surface restored in a tooth colored material.
8	**M (mesial) caries.** The area of decay is outlined.
9	**Fracture.** A jagged line indicates the area of fracture.
13	**Full crown, porcelain fused to metal crown.** In the mouth this crown appears to be all tooth colored.
16	**To be extracted.** Parallel lines indicate a tooth which must be extracted.
17	**Impacted.** The tooth is circled to show impaction. An arrow is used to indicate the direction of drift.
19	**OF (occlusal and facial) caries.** The area of decay is outlined.
20	**MOD (mesial, occlusal, distal) amalgam restoration.** The restored area is filled in using ink.
24	**Completed RCT.** A line through the root area indicates endodontic treatment.
25	**Abscess.** A circle at the root tip indicates a periapical abscess.
30	**DO (distal, occlusal) amalgam restoration.** The restored area is filled in using ink.
31	**MO (mesial, occlusal) caries.** The area of decay is outlined.
32	**Missing.**

Figure 4-8. Charting symbols and explanations.

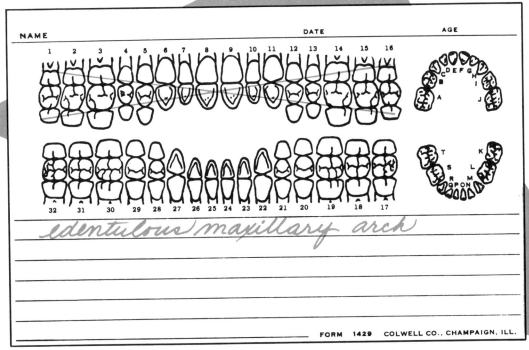

Figure 4-9. An exam sheet used to chart a recall examination.

Examination Slips

Examination slips are a short form with a charting diagram and space for remarks (Fig. 4-9). These slips are frequently used at recall visits to chart the findings from the patient's most recent examination.

TREATMENT ABBREVIATIONS			
Anes	Local anesthetic	FT	Fluoride treatment
Adj	Adjustment	GR	Gold restoration
Amal	Amalgam restoration	GT	Gingival treatment
BA	Broken appointment	NC	no charge
BWX	Bite-wing x-rays	PA	Preparatory appointment
CA	Corrective appliance	Partial	Partial denture
C & B	Crown and bridge	POT	Post operative treatment
Comp	Composite restoration	Prophy	Prophylaxis
DR	Denture repair	RCT	Root canal therapy
DS	Denture service	SR 1, 2, 3	Surfaces restored
Ext	Extraction	ST	Sedative treatment
Exam	Examination	SM	Study models
FMX	Full mouth x-rays	X	X-ray(s)

SERVICE ENTRIES

Entries in the "service rendered" portion of the chart note are always made in ink. Each entry should include the date, tooth number and surfaces involved, and an exact listing of the service rendered including details such as materials used.

▶ Treatment Abbreviations

Each dentist has abbreviations that he or she uses to record these service entries. The Table *"Treatment Abbreviations"* shows samples of commonly used abbreviations.

▶ When in doubt, write it out.

When working with abbreviations, it is important to be clear on the meaning of each abbreviation used. Don't take chances. If in doubt, write it out.

The abbreviations used for recording treatment on a chart are not necessarily the same as those which will be used in the bookkeeping system to record charges. Shown here are sample chart entries to record the treatment provided.

Date	Tooth	Service
1/05/XX		*Exam, prophy, 4 BWX*

Shown above is the entry for an examination, prophylaxis and four bite-wing x-rays.

Date	Tooth	Service
1/20/XX	14 MO	*Anes, dycal, amal*

Shown above is the entry for the placement of a two-surface mesial-occlusal (MO) amalgam restoration in tooth #14. Local anesthetic solution was administered and Dycal (a cavity liner) was placed under the restoration.

Date	Tooth	Service
3/10/XX	32	*X, anes, ext*

Shown above is the entry for an x-ray, local anesthesia and the extraction of tooth #32.

▶ Charting Errors

▶ If you make a charting error, take the steps necessary to correct it properly.

If an error is made when entering a service rendered, never try to cover it up or to erase it. Instead, follow the proper procedure for correcting it.

- Draw a line through the error, but do not block the entry so it can't be read.
- Make the corrected entry on the next available line.
- Initial and date the changes.

▶ **Entering Fees**

Although many charts include a space to note fees, it is <u>not</u> a good idea to keep the account financial records here. There are two reasons for this.

✓ **First,** the patient's chart is a clinical record and as such is not the place for financial information.

✓ **Second,** financial records can be managed more effectively when they are organized in one place, such as on a ledger card or account history.

▶ Fees are <u>not</u> entered on the patient's chart.

Chapter

PREVENTIVE RECALL AND WRITTEN COMMUNICATIONS

LEARNING GOALS

The student will be able to:

▶ List at least four services that are included in a recall visit.
▶ Describe at least three types of recall systems.
▶ Discuss how the use of greeting cards is a practice building tool.
▶ Demonstrate calculating the month of recall for a patient.
▶ Demonstrate writing a "welcome to our practice" letter in a block format.
▶ Demonstrate addressing a ledger card or other correspondence correctly.

OVERVIEW OF RECALL SYSTEMS

Recall is the process of periodically reminding patients that it is time to return to the practice for a check-up visit or for follow-up care.

Recall is a service offered to patients because the dentist believes they need this care. Also, because of the ongoing patient flow that it generates, recall can be important to the economic health of the practice.

▶ Recall Is More Than Just A Cleaning

▶ Recall is more than just a cleaning.

Most patients think a recall appointment is a visit just to have their teeth cleaned. And from the patient's point of view, a routine cleaning can easily be postponed indefinitely. Actually at each recall visit many services are provided including:

✓ Oral cancer screening.
✓ Thorough examination of the hard and soft tissues of the mouth to detect any developing pathology.
✓ Home care review and reinforcement.
✓ Follow-up care for previously completed treatment such as endodontic treatment or crown and bridge.
✓ For children, the early detection of any developmental problems.

▶ Recall Is Patient Education

A successful recall program begins with patient education, because patients who fail to realize the importance of this preventive care are not likely to return regularly for their recall visits.

You can help by making patients aware of the benefits of recall and by assisting them in making and keeping their recall appointments.

PLACING THE PATIENT ON RECALL

The point at which the patient's name is entered into the recall system depends upon the dentist's policy. In some practices this is done when the patient completes his current series of dental treatments. In other practices it is at the time of the patient's prophy (cleaning).

▶ Calculating The Recall Period

No matter what type of recall system is used, the steps necessary to place the patient on recall should be completed before the patient's records are filed.

The time span between recall visits is determined by the dentist based on the patient's needs; however, a six-month period is the time frame used most frequently.

The Table *"Calculating The Recall Date"* helps in determining when the patient should be notified to return.

- To calculate a six-month recall in the first half of the year, just add six to the number of the month.
- For months in the last half of the year, subtract six.
- To calculate any other recall period count ahead the desired number of months.

CALCULATING THE RECALL DATE					
1	2	3	4	5	6
JAN	FEB	MARCH	APRIL	MAY	JUNE
JULY	AUG	SEPT	OCT	NOV	DEC
7	8	9	10	11	12

 Processing Recall Notices

Recall notices for the following month are usually handled around the middle of the month. This helps to equalize the workload throughout the month and eases the "end-of-the-month rush" which may result when statements and recalls must be prepared and mailed at the same time.

METHODS OF NOTIFYING RECALL PATIENTS

The kind of recall system used will depend to a large extent on the method used to notify patients. This may be by telephone, mail, or a combination of telephone and mail.

 Telephone Recall Reminder

Notifying recall patients by telephone is time-consuming; however, it has the advantage that once contact has been made the patient will often set up the recall appointment.

 Mailed Recall Reminders

Mailed reminders have the advantages of being faster and easier to process. This recall method has the disadvantage that it is then up to the patient to be sufficiently motivated to call and make the appointment.

Mailed notices work particularly well for practices where there are many patients to be notified each month. These reminders are usually either a postcard or greeting card type (Fig. 5-1).

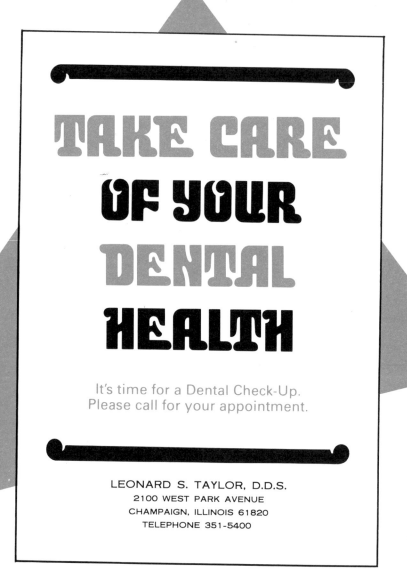

Figure 5-1. Recall reminder card to be mailed to the patient.

COMPUTERIZED RECALL SYSTEMS

A computerized bookkeeping system usually includes a function to manage the recall system. Most systems offer flexibility in that they can:

- Address postcard type recall cards.
- Print mailing labels or address envelopes for recall cards.
- Generate personalized letters as written reminders.
- Create a list of names, phone numbers and reason-for-recall to be used for telephone reminders (Fig. 5-2).
- Make it possible to track, and follow-up on, those patients who fail to respond to the recall notices.

```
         RECALL  BY  TELEPHONE     Leonard  S.  Taylor,  D.D.S.

         MEMBER/                    AGE/   LAST   ***RECALL***
ACCOUNT  HOME AND WORK TELEPHONE    SEX    VISIT  MONTHS DATE

    4    William    Phillips        68 01-03-       6 07-03-
         356-4421                    M

    9    Martin     Hall            46 01-21-       6 07-21-
         351-8142        344-1782    M

    9    Paul       Peterson         6 01-10-       6 07-10-
         351-8142        344-1782    M

   18    Charles    Baker           40 01-28-       6 07-21-
         551-2401        882-3489    M

   18    Lisa       Baker            8 01-03-       6 07-03-
         551-2401        882-3489    F

   18    David      Baker           14 01-21-       6 07-21-
         551-2401        882-3489    M

   23    Cynthia    Nelson           7 01-10-       6 07-10-
         882-0029        541-9721    F

   44    Laurie     Brown           32 01-21-       6 07-21-
         367-4781                    F

   46    Nancy      Moore           29 01-10-       6 07-10-
         882-5678                    F

   55    Barry      Nolan           27 01-21-       6 07-21-
         844-7653        884-3639    M

   59    Dean       Randle          32 01-21-       6 07-21-
                                     M

   65    Theodore   Rockwell        26 01-10-       6 07-10-
         882-5241                    M

   66    Wallace    Pierce          58 01-11-       6 07-03-
         844-6310                    M
```

Figure 5-2. A computer generated recall list.

OTHER TYPES OF RECALL SYSTEMS

▶ Advance Appointment System

The advance appointment system, also known as the *continuing appointment system,* is based on making a definite recall appointment for the patient at the time of his last visit in the current series. The date and time are verified with the patient and he is given an appointment card.

This system has the advantage that the patient is committed to return for this visit and his return does not depend entirely upon his motivation six months hence. It has the disadvantage that these appointments are frequently broken, changed or cancelled.

These recall appointments are coded in the appointment book so that the patient may be sent a reminder card two weeks before the date (Fig. 5-3). These appointments should also be confirmed by telephone several days prior to the scheduled time.

▶ List-By-Month Recall System

A list is most effective in an office where recall patients are reminded by telephone. With this system a list is made, by the month, of patients scheduled to be recalled in that month.

This list is usually kept on the computer or in the back of the appointment book. When the patient's name is added to the list, his telephone number is noted next to it so that he may be contacted by phone.

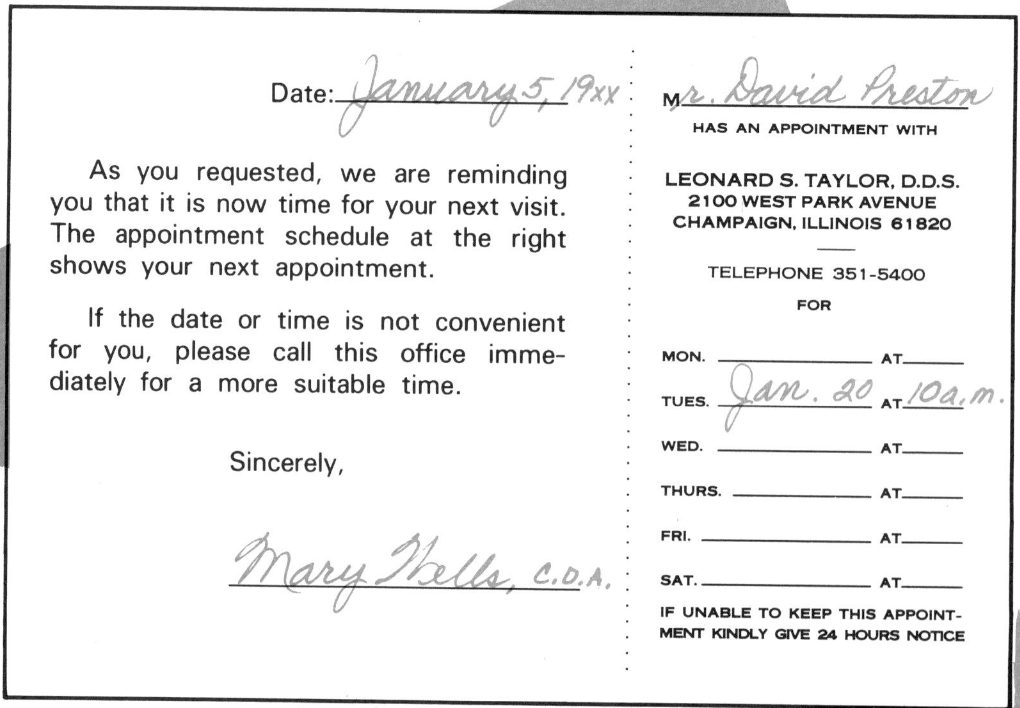

Date: *January 5, 19xx*

Mr. *David Preston*

HAS AN APPOINTMENT WITH

LEONARD S. TAYLOR, D.D.S.
2100 WEST PARK AVENUE
CHAMPAIGN, ILLINOIS 61820

TELEPHONE 351-5400

FOR

MON. _____ AT_____

TUES. *Jan. 20* AT *10 a.m.*

WED. _____ AT_____

THURS. _____ AT_____

FRI. _____ AT_____

SAT. _____ AT_____

IF UNABLE TO KEEP THIS APPOINTMENT KINDLY GIVE 24 HOURS NOTICE

As you requested, we are reminding you that it is now time for your next visit. The appointment schedule at the right shows your next appointment.

If the date or time is not convenient for you, please call this office immediately for a more suitable time.

Sincerely,

Mary Wells, C.O.A.

Figure 5-3. A postcard reminder for a patient who has made an advance recall appointment.

▶ **Recall Tracking System**

The recall tracking system makes it possible to maintain an on-going record of the patient's response to recall reminders (Fig. 5-4).

With this system, the recall tracking card is completed the first time the patient is placed on recall. There is space on the card for the:

- Patient's name and address.
- Home and work telephone numbers.
- Dates of recall notices and the patient's responses.
- Reason for recall or other notes.

| JAN | FEB | MAR | APR | MAY | JUN | JUL | AUG | SEP | OCT | NOV | DEC |

NAME OF PATIENT *David Preston*		NAME OF SPOUSE/PARENT *Harold Preston*	
HOME ADDRESS *4456 Terrace Drive, Champaign, Il 61820*			HOME PHONE *432-5312*
EMPLOYER	BUSINESS ADDRESS		BUSINESS PHONE

RECALL DATE(S)			RESPONSE DATE	APPOINTMENT DATE	NOTES
6/xx			6/25/xx	7/7/xx	*check sealants*
2/xx			4/1/xx	4/13/xx	*fluoride treatment*
10/xx					*prophy*

Form 1050 Colwell Systems, Inc., Champaign, IL 61820

Figure 5-4. Sample recall tracking card.

The card is completed the first time the patient is placed on recall. At that time it is tagged with a colored metal file signal to indicate the month of recall, and is filed alphabetically.

Because the cards are filed alphabetically, instead of by dates, filing is faster. It is also easier to look up recall information for a patient or family.

When it is time to process recall notices, those cards tagged for recall that month are removed from the file and the file signals are removed for reuse.

If patients are being **notified by telephone**, the results of the phone calls are noted on the card. When the telephone notification is complete, the results are noted and the card is returned to the file.

If patients are being **notified by mail**, the recall card envelopes are addressed using information from the recall tracking card. The date of recall notification is noted on the card and the tracking card is returned to the alphabetical file.

When it is time to place the patient on recall again, the same card is reused by simply placing a colored metal file signal to indicate the new month of recall.

▶ The Combination Recall System

The combination recall system is also known as the *Complete Recall System*. This system combines sending written notices and then using the telephone to follow up on those patients who fail to respond. It is based on the use of:

✓ A three-part NCR (no carbon required) recall form (Fig. 5-5).
✓ A chronological file that divides each month into two sections: 1 through 15 and 16 through 31.
✓ An alphabetical file for cards waiting to be reused.

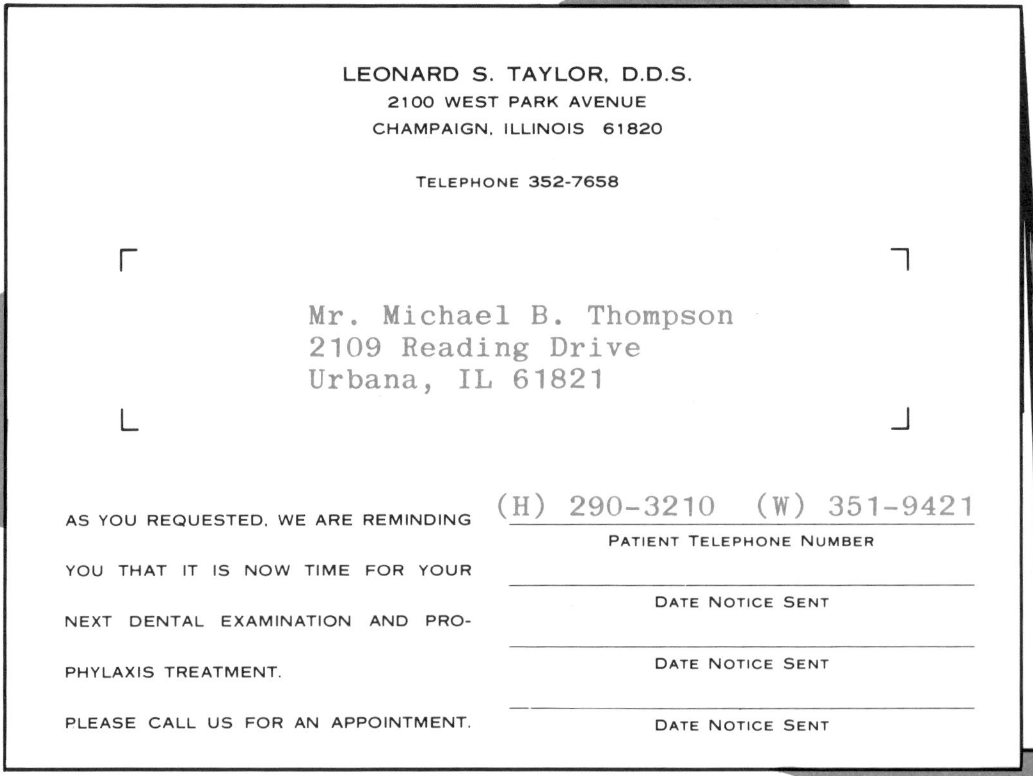

LEONARD S. TAYLOR, D.D.S.
2100 WEST PARK AVENUE
CHAMPAIGN, ILLINOIS 61820

TELEPHONE 352-7658

Mr. Michael B. Thompson
2109 Reading Drive
Urbana, IL 61821

AS YOU REQUESTED, WE ARE REMINDING YOU THAT IT IS NOW TIME FOR YOUR NEXT DENTAL EXAMINATION AND PROPHYLAXIS TREATMENT. PLEASE CALL US FOR AN APPOINTMENT.

(H) 290-3210 (W) 351-9421
PATIENT TELEPHONE NUMBER

DATE NOTICE SENT

DATE NOTICE SENT

DATE NOTICE SENT

Figure 5-5. Sample 3-part combination recall card.

Placing The Patient On Recall

1. When it is time to place the patient on recall, have the patient complete the form for himself. One writing completes all three copies.

2. The form is filed alphabetically in a chronological file in the first section (1 through 15) for the month of recall.

Processing The Notices

1. When it is time to process recall notices, remove the form from the file and note the date of the first notification.

2. Place the top copy of the form in a window envelope and mail it to the patient.

3. Move the remaining copies ahead to the second section (16 through 31) for the month of recall.

4. When the patient responds, remove the remaining copies from this file and place them in an alphabetical file. These may be reused the next time the patient is placed on recall.

The Second Notice

1. After the 15th of the month, remove the cards from the second section of the file.

2. Date the second notification and mail the top copy to the patient as a second reminder.

3. Return the remaining copy to the chronological file.

Following Up

1. At the beginning of the next month, review the cards still remaining in the second section of the previous month.

2. For those patients who still have not responded, you have several choices. You may:

   * Send the third written notice.

   * Telephone the patient to set up an appointment.

   * Remove the notice and do not contact the patient again.

RECALL TELEPHONE CALLS

The process of notifying recall patients by telephone should be started around the middle of the month. Doing this helps to equalize the workload through the month. Because this process is time consuming, some practices divide the recall list into four groups and contact one group each week. The following are guidelines for making these calls.

 Space The Calls

Do not make the calls one right after another. This ties up the phone lines, and patients trying to reach you will get busy signals. Instead, space out the calls or make them on a day when the office is closed.

 Be Enthusiastic

Greet the patient with enthusiasm and a cheerful message. For example, *"Mrs. Thomas, we are looking forward to seeing you again."*

Remind the patient of the importance of the recall visit. For example, *"As you remember Mrs. Thomas, Dr. Taylor said he wanted to check those new bonded veneers in six months."*

▶ Be Prepared To Offer Choices

If you ask the patient, *"Would you like to make an appointment now?"*, the answer is likely to be *"No."*

If you ask the patient, *"Which would be more convenient for you, Monday the 25th at 2:30 or Wednesday the 27th at 9 a.m.?"* it is more difficult for him to say no.

▶ Record The Results

Always note the results of the call on the patient's recall record. In addition to recording the date on which you reached the patient, also note:

✓ If the patient made an appointment, note the date of that appointment.

✓ If the patient did not make an appointment, note this and the date when a follow-up call would be appropriate.

✓ If the patient asked that you not call again, note this and inform the dentist. There may be a problem here with a dissatisfied patient.

GREETING CARDS

▶ Patients appreciate receiving mail from the doctor's office other than a bill!

Patients appreciate receiving mail from the doctor's office that is something other than a bill! The thoughtful use of greeting cards is an effective way to market the practice and to let patients know that the doctor really does care about them!

There are cards available that are designed specifically for use by professional practices. These can be purchased printed with the doctor's name; however, a signature adds a much more personal touch.

- Children and the elderly particularly like receiving **birthday cards.**
- New parents appreciate **congratulations cards.**
- Everyone enjoys receiving seasonal greetings such as **Christmas** or other appropriate **holiday cards.**
- A carefully selected **sympathy card** expresses sensitivity and lets the family know that the doctor shares their sense of loss.

▶ Sending Birthday Cards

In order to send birthday cards with a minimum of fuss, you need to establish a system. If you are using a computerized bookkeeping system, it should generate a list of patients who are having birthdays each month. The system should also generate mailing labels for these cards.

If you are not using a computer you can make the recall tracking system serve double duty. To do this:

1. Note the patient's date of birth on the recall tracking card. Add a second color coded signal to indicate the month of birth.

2. Prior to the beginning of the month, pull the cards for patients having a birthday in the next month. Do <u>not</u> remove the color file signal indicating the month of birth.

3. Prepare the birthday cards and envelopes. On the envelope, where the stamp will be placed, note the date of the birthday. Then, arrange the prepared cards into weekly groups based on the date of the birthday.

4. Return the record cards to their place in the alphabetical file. Take care not to disturb the colored file signal indicating the month of recall.

5. Mail the cards in weekly batches so that the card will reach the patient near his birthday.

COMPUTERIZED WORD PROCESSING

The use of a word processor or electronic typewriter makes it possible to generate a letter without typing or spelling errors. It also makes it easier to determine that the letter is positioned correctly on the page.

✓ If using "spell check" on a computer, add frequently used technical terms to the "master list" in the system.

✓ Always "spell check" a document before the final printing.

✓ Also, review your copy very carefully to identify errors such as using the wrong term or an incorrect tense. (The computer can't catch these.)

LETTER WRITING

All correspondence that leaves the office must be neat, clean, properly placed on the page and professional in appearance (Fig. 5-6).

The text of the letter must be simply worded and free of spelling, typing or grammatical errors.

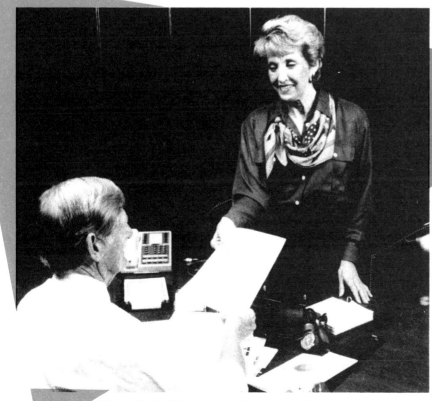

Figure 5-6. All correspondence must be neat and professional in appearance.

The five steps below will help you write better letters. After you've written a letter, read it over and check it against the guidelines found in the Table "*How Do Your Letters Rate?*"

Step #1 — Plan Ahead

Be certain that your letter says exactly what you mean it to say. To accomplish this, you should:

- List the points you want to make.
- Arrange them in logical sequence.
- Then write your letter so that these points are clearly made.

Step #2 — Keep It Simple

Do not use difficult words when short, simple ones will do. Also, do not use long complex sentences or flowery language when a plain statement would be easier to understand.

Step #3 — Avoid Unnecessary Professional Jargon

As you learn the language of dentistry don't forget that not everyone understands it — and that the terms can be very confusing. Whenever possible, select words you are certain the patient can understand.

However, if you are writing a consultation report to another professional, it is necessary to include all of the technical terms (as dictated by the doctor). If in doubt, double check that you have used and spelled the terms correctly.

Step #4 — Check Your Spelling

▶ Spelling always counts.

A misspelled word can greatly change the meaning of the sentence. Therefore, spelling always counts!

All words, particularly technical terms, must be spelled correctly. Even if you are using a word processing program with "spell check," keep a dictionary near your desk and refer to it as often as necessary to be sure that your spelling is correct.

Step #5 — Select The Style

Today most letters are written in a **block style** in which all parts of the letter start at the left margin (Figs. 5-7 & 5-8).

Some doctors prefer a **modified block style.** Here the date line is centered two lines below the last line of the letterhead, and the complimentary close and signature begin five spaces to the left of the center of the page.

ADDRESSING OUTGOING MAIL

It is important that outgoing mail be addressed correctly. This includes: ledger cards (which will be photocopied as monthly statements), insurance claims, recall notices, letters and all correspondence. The following are the guidelines recommended by the United State Postal Service (Fig. 5-9).

HOW DO YOUR LETTERS RATE?	
✓	**Appearance**
	Does the letter's appearance make a good first impression?
	Is it well-balanced on the page?
	Are the paragraphs short enough to invite easy reading?
	Has it been checked for errors in grammar and punctuation?
	Has it been checked for spelling errors?
✓	**Effectiveness**
	Does it achieve your goal in writing the letter?
	Does it include all the information the reader needs?
	Is the material presented in logical order?
	Is it clear, concise, and readable?
	Is it visually inviting to the reader?
✓	**Attitude**
	Does it sound as if one human being has written it to another?
	Does it avoid technical jargon?
	Have you eliminated trite, meaningless, or wordy expressions?
	Is it friendly, courteous, tactful, and sincere?
	Does it build good will?

The Attention Line

The first line of the address is called the attention line. This is the name of the person to whom the letter is being sent.

When addressing mail to a business, such as an insurance company or supplier, that information goes on the next line.

The Address Line

Next is the address line which includes the street address, post office box number, or rural route number. On this line, also include:

- **Building number and street name.**
- **Direction guidelines** are abbreviated as: N (north), S (south), E (east), W (west)
- **Street designations** are abbreviated as: AVE (avenue), ST (street), DR (drive), RD (road), PL (place), CIR (circle)
- **Exact location designations** are abbreviated as: RM (room), STE (suite), APT (apartment number)

In their recommendations, the postal service does <u>not</u> place punctuation between the street address and exact location designations.

▶ The City, State And Zip Code Line

The final line of the address is the name of the city and state plus the zip code.

✓ Use the two letter abbreviation for the state
✓ If you know the full code (zip+4), use it.

In their recommendations, the postal service does <u>not</u> place punctuation between the city, state and zip code.

Leonard S. Taylor, D.D.S.
2100 W Park Ave
Champaign IL 61820

MR ROBERT CLAWSON
ACME REPAIR SERVICE
2000 PEACHTREE ST NE STE 410
ATLANTA GA 30340-4421

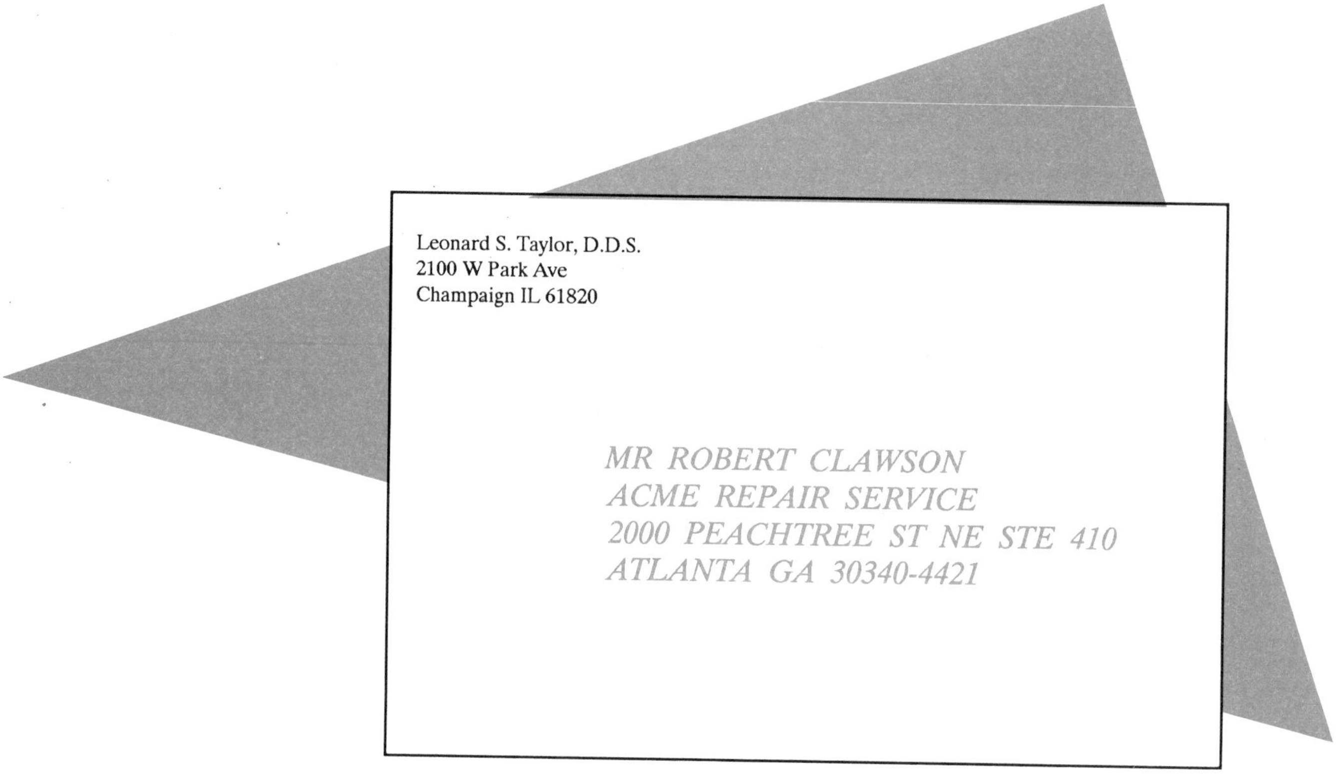

Figure 5-9. Envelope addressed according to U.S. Postal Service guidelines.

LEONARD S. TAYLOR, D.D.S.

Date	March 5, 19XX
Inside address	Margo Henderson, D.D.S. 5519 Broad Street Champaign, IL 61820
Salutation	Dear Dr. Henderson:
Body of letter	Thank you for referring Alex Jackson to me for treatment. It was a pleasure meeting Alex and his parents. In my examination of Alex I found rampant caries which will require extractions, amalgam restorations and stainless crowns. Because of Alex's severe mental retardation, treatment must be performed under general anesthesia. Alex is scheduled for treatment at Champaign Memorial Hospital on March 15, 19XX. Soon thereafter I will send you a full report.
Complimentary close	Sincerely,
Signature	*Leonard S. Taylor, D.D.S.* Leonard S. Taylor, D.D.S.
Reference initials	LST/mw
Carbon copies	cc: Mr. and Mrs. Jackson

2100 WEST PARK AVENUE   CHAMPAIGN, ILLINOIS 61820   TELEPHONE 351-5400

Figure 5-7. Sample letter to a referring dentist (in block format).

LEONARD S. TAYLOR, D.D.S.

March 5, 19XX

Mrs. Robert Olson
2300 Maple Street
Champaign, IL 61820

Dear Mrs. Olson:

Our records show that it has been more than a year since Kathy and Kevin were in for their dental checkups.

Regular preventive care is very important for children because it enables us to protect their dental health. Also, if developmental problems are detected early we are able to correct many of them before major treatment is required.

For your convenience, we now have expanded Saturday hours. Please phone today for an appointment.

Sincerely,

Mary Wells, C.D.A.

Mary Wells, C.D.A.,
Secretarial Assistant to
Leonard S. Taylor, D.D.S.

2100 WEST PARK AVENUE   CHAMPAIGN, ILLINOIS   61820   TELEPHONE 351-5400

Figure 5-8. Sample recall letter (in block format).

Chapter

ACCOUNTS
RECEIVABLE
BOOKKEEPING

LEARNING GOALS

The student will be able to:

▶ Define accounts receivable bookkeeping, transactions and posting.
▶ State the type of information that the patient needs, and that which the practice requires.
▶ List the five parts of an accounts receivable bookkeeping system and state the purpose of each.
▶ Describe the use of charge slips as part of the audit trail.
▶ Demonstrate entering charges, payments and adjustments on a pegboard bookkeeping system.
▶ Describe how these functions would be managed on a computerized system.
▶ Demonstrate making specialized account entries and adjustments.
▶ Describe the steps in preparing a bank deposit.

OVERVIEW OF ACCOUNTS RECEIVABLE BOOKKEEPING

▶ Accounts receivable bookkeeping is the recording and management of all patient account transactions within the practice.

Accounts receivable bookkeeping is the recording and management of all patient account transactions within the practice. Accounts receivable bookkeeping is not difficult; however, it does require accuracy and careful attention to detail. Also, these duties must be managed in a timely and business-like manner so that all of the appropriate records are accurate and current.

▶ Financial Transactions

A **transaction** is any financial entry made to an account record. The three types of transactions are:

- A **charge** which increases the account balance.
- A **payment** which decreases the account balance.
- An **adjustment** which may increase or decrease the account balance.

▶ Posting

Posting is the act of entering transaction information into the bookkeeping system. The use of codes to speed posting is explained later in this chapter.

▶ Bookkeeping Information Requirements

The accounts receivable bookkeeping system must generate records to fill two types of data requirements. These are the information needs of the patient and the information needs of the practice.

Patient Information

The patient must have information about his account so that he may meet his financial obligations to the practice. He needs to know:

1. What services were provided and how much was charged.

2. How much has been paid on the account.

3. The amount of the current balance on the account.

As a service to the patient, this account record information is provided to him in the form of a:

✓ Receipt or walk-out statement at the time of his visit.
✓ Monthly statement.
✓ Completed insurance claim.

Practice Information

The practice needs to know how much is owed on each account. However, the practice also requires summaries of total financial activities and amounts owed, management reports and an audit trail.

These records must provide the data necessary to operate the practice in a business-like manner, and to meet government recordkeeping requirements.

THE PARTS OF A BOOKKEEPING SYSTEM

In a dental practice, accounts receivable bookkeeping is usually managed using either a manual system, such as a one-write pegboard, or with a computerized system.

Both systems include the same five major parts which are compared on the Table *"Comparing Manual And Computerized Bookkeeping Systems."* These parts are:

#1 — Patient account records

#2 — Charge slips

#3 — Receipts and walk-out statements

#4 — Management reports

#5 — An audit trail

COMPARING MANUAL AND COMPUTERIZED BOOKKEEPING SYSTEMS		
System Part	**Manual System**	**Computerized system**
Account records	Maintained on paper **ledger cards.**	Organized in files called **account histories.**
Charge slips	Completed manually on the pegboard.	Generated by the computer <u>or</u> completed manually.
Receipts / Walk-out statements	Completed manually as transactions are posted.	Generated by the computer <u>or</u> completed manually.
Management reports	Completed manually.	Generated by the computer.
Audit trail	Must be maintained by the user.	Must be maintained by the user.

 #1 — Patient Account Records

Patient account records contain data concerning all account transactions plus the current balance owed on the account. Account records are usually maintained by family, and the record is always addressed to the person responsible for payment of that account (Fig. 6-1).

#2 — Charge Slips

A charge slip is used to transmit account information from the business office to the treatment area and back again to the business office. Without this flow of information, it is impossible to accurately capture all fees and patient charges.

Charge slips, which are used with both computerized and manual systems, are also known as:

- **encounter forms,**
- **routing slips,**
- **superbills,** and
- **transmittal documents.**

LEONARD S. TAYLOR, D.D.S.
2100 WEST PARK AVENUE
CHAMPAIGN, ILLINOIS 61822

TELEPHONE 367-6671

Mr. James A. Gridley
670 Northridge Terrace
Champaign, IL 61820

DATE	FAMILY MEMBER	PROFESSIONAL SERVICE	CHARGE	CREDITS PAYM'TS	ADJ	BALANCE
1/2/xx		BALANCE FORWARD				$25.00
1/9/xx	James	SR S2	45 00	25 00		45 00
1/15/xx	Ruth	GT	125 00			170 00
2/10/xx		ck		170 00		-0-

1625

PAY LAST AMOUNT IN THIS COLUMN ⌂

O - OFFICE CALL	SR - SILVER RESTORATION	DS - DENTURE SERVICE
X - X-RAYS	GR - GOLD RESTORATION	GT - GINGIVAL TREATMENT
E - EXTRACTION	PR - PORCELAIN RESTORATION	CA - CORRECTIVE APPLIANCE
P - PROPHYLAXIS	OS - ORAL SURGERY	RP - REPARATIVE PROCEDURE
S - SEDATIVE TREATMENT	CB - CROWN OR BRIDGE SERVICE	PA - PREPARATORY APPOINTMENT

Figure 6-1. Sample account ledger card.

Guidelines For Using Charge Slips

1. Charge slips are an important part of the audit trail. Numbered charge slips should be used and each number must be accounted for.

2. A charge slip must be prepared for every patient (even if this is a "no charge" visit).

3. The prepared charge slip shows the account name and current balance.

   This information is provided so that if there is a problem with an over-due or very large balance, the dentist will be aware of it.

4. The charge slip is sent into the treatment area with the patient's chart. At the end of the patient's visit the dentist or assistant notes on the charge slip the services and fees for the current visit.

5. When the charge slip is returned to the business office, the charges are entered into the bookkeeping system and the patient is asked for payment.

 #3 — Receipts And Walk-Out Statements

A patient must always be given a receipt for a cash payment. If the account is not paid in full, the patient is given a "walk-out statement" showing the current balance on the account.

 The patient is always given a receipt for a cash payment.

With the walk-out statement, the patient receives a reply envelope and is asked to mail the payment as soon as possible. This speeds collections and reduces the number of statements which must be sent at the end of the month.

With a manual system, this is generated as the entries are made in the bookkeeping system. With a computerized system, there is usually the option of printing a receipt or walk-out statement form.

 #4 — Management Reports

The reports generated by the bookkeeping system provide essential information for the management of the practice.

The Daily Journal Record

Patient account records maintain the records of individual account activity. The daily journal ties together these individual records and forms a summary of all practice activity on a day-to-day basis (Fig. 6-2). This includes a record of:

- **Total production** of all services provided. This shows the services rendered and fees charged for each patient seen throughout the day.
- **Payments received** each business day. The total receipts amount shown on the daily journal record should match exactly the total amount deposited for the day.
- **Adjustments,** which may increase or decrease the amount of the account balance. These are also listed here.
- **Balances outstanding,** which shows the current amount owed on the account.
- **Accounts receivable totals,** which is the total of all outstanding balances owed to the practice.

```
        01-11-      DAILY LOG   Leonard S. Taylor, D.D.S.

ACCOUNT      DESCRIPTION        CHARGE      PAID    ADJ.    BALANCE  PATIEN
```

ACCOUNT	DESCRIPTION	CHARGE	PAID	ADJ.	BALANCE	PATIEN
2	Mr. Harry Cummins					
	Insurance Payment		67.00		0.00	
12	Mrs. Janice Martin-Jones					
	Prophylaxis, Adult	20.00			148.78	Janice
	4 Bitewing X-Rays	16.00			164.78	Janice
	Personal Check		36.00		128.78	
15	Mr. Vincent Montgomery					
	Insurance Payment		71.00		0.00	
23	Mr. Greg Nelson					
	C & B Gold Crown	300.00			363.00	Doroth
	Bridge Pontic	300.00			663.00	Doroth
	C & B Porcelain	300.00			963.00	Doroth
	Personal Check		500.00		463.00	
31	Ms. Ruth Green					
	RCT, Single Canal	125.00			213.00	Ruth
33	Mr. Lawrence Porter					
	Occ. Adjustment	40.00			129.63	Susan
	Cash		50.00		79.63	
50	Miss Lisa Norman					
	Amalgam, 3 Surf.	36.00			119.74	Lisa
	Amalgam, 2 Surf.	28.00			147.74	Lisa
	Personal Check		83.74		64.00	
51	Mr. Edward Colson					
	Initial Oral Exam	12.00			101.00	Faye
	Sedative Filling	10.00			111.00	Faye
	Credit Card		111.00		0.00	
61	Mr. Albert Newton					
	Amalgam, 1 Surf.	20.00			101.00	Frances
66	Wallace Pierce					
	Comp. Upper Denture	325.00			587.33	Wallace
	Personal Check		300.00		287.33	
68	Charles French					
	Insurance Payment		288.30		61.70	
	Insurance Adjustment			21.70-	40.00	
70	Mr. Lionel Agnew					
	Post Op Treatment	0.00			49.45	Lionel
	Cash		25.00		24.45	
71	Mrs. Andrew Dawson					
	BCBS Payment		128.75		27.56	

```
 Leonard S. Taylor, D.D.S.    1532.00   1660.79   21.70-
                              -------   -------   -------
                     TOTALS   1532.00   1660.79   21.70-

                     CASH                  75.00
                     CHECK               1474.79
                     CREDIT CARD          111.00
```

Figure 6-2. Computer generated daily summary report.

Monthly Statements

Monthly statements are sent to all patient accounts with outstanding balances. Statements are discussed in Chapter 8.

Monthly And Annual Summaries

The totals from the daily journal records are carried forward to monthly and annual summaries which show the total of all earnings and income for the practice.

Based on the summary data, the Accounts Receivable report and other management reports are generated. With a manual system, these reports can be generated using special forms. With a computer, these reports are automatically generated by the system.

▶ #5 — The Audit Trail

The audit trail is an important part of every accounts receivable system because it is the means of making certain that all bookkeeping entries are being made accurately and honestly.

▶ The audit trail is the means of determining that all bookkeeping entries are being made accurately and honestly.

Maintaining the audit trail enables an honest employee to detect errors, and protects the employer against embezzlement by a dishonest employee. (**Embezzlement** is the illegal act of stealing practice funds by manipulating the bookkeeping records.) The basic elements of an audit trail include:

Accounting For Each Patient Visit

The numbered charge slips are used for this purpose, and at the end of the day, each charge slip must be accounted for.

Some computerized systems generate numbered charge slips. Then, at the end of the day, the system prints a report noting any charge slips that were not accounted for. With a manual system, it is necessary to review the charge slip numbers shown on the daily journal page.

When a charge slip is missing, it indicates that there may be a problem and that patient charges were not posted to the system. Missing slips should be tracked promptly and accounted for.

Daily Deposit Of All Receipts

At the end of the day, the amount of checks and cash in the drawer should match exactly the total receipts shown on the daily journal page. (This is after the amount of the cash fund has been removed.) All receipts are then deposited daily.

Periodic Spot Checks

In order for an audit trail to be effective, the dentist must remain involved in the process. This includes making periodic and random spot checks to determine that all bookkeeping entries are being made accurately.

THE CHANGE FUND

It is a courtesy to have change available for a patient who wishes to make a cash payment. The change fund is a supply of cash, usually $100 or less in small bills, which is maintained for this purpose.

The money for the change fund is placed in the cash drawer at the beginning of the day and used throughout the day. At the end of the day, before the bank deposit is prepared, the exact amount of the change fund is removed to a safe place (to be used again the next day).

Occasionally a patient will offer to pay by writing a check for more than the amount due — and then expect "change" in cash.

Although doing this seems to be a service to the patient, it could create problems for the practice.

✓ First, it depletes the cash fund.
✓ Second, if the check does not clear the bank, the practice is out the amount of the visit plus the amount of cash given as "change."
✓ Third, it confuses the practice records and the patient's personal records as to exactly how much was paid to the doctor.

PEGBOARD BOOKKEEPING

> Pegboard is the most widely used manual bookkeeping system for dental practices.

Pegboard is the most widely used manual bookkeeping system for dental practices. With it, all the necessary records are completed in a single writing. This assures that all records are the same and that no entries are omitted. The following elements work together to make this possible (Fig. 6-3).

 ### The Pegboard

The pegboard is so named because it has a row of pegs projecting along the left side of the board. The accounting forms fit over these pegs and are aligned so that writing on the top form will transfer through to the forms beneath.

 ### The Daily Journal

The daily journal, also known as the "*Daily Log of Charges and Receipts*," has holes along the left edge to fit on the pegs of the pegboard.

Ledger Cards

Account histories are maintained on ledger cards printed with lines and columns that exactly match those on the daily journal page (and on the receipt and charge slips).

These cards are printed on special NCR (no carbon required) paper so that entries transfer through the card and onto the daily journal page.

Ledger cards are stored alphabetically in a ledger card file tray. When in use, the cards are fully visible and easily accessible. When not in use, the cards are compacted tightly together to provide some protection against fire.

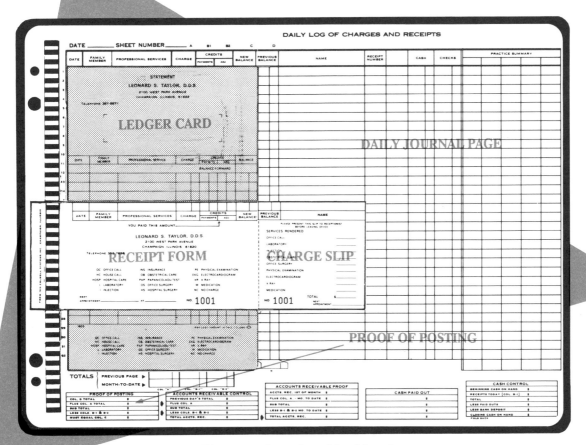

Figure 6-3. Elements of a pegboard bookkeeping system.

► Receipt And Charge Slips

These forms are numbered and are made up of two parts. The right end serves as a charge slip. The left portion is a receipt (Fig. 6-4).

They come shingled in banks of 25, and also fit the pegs on the left side of the board.

Receipt and charge slips have a carbon strip along the back of the top edge so that entries also appear on the account ledger card and are transferred through to the daily journal page.

These forms, and the account ledger cards, are printed with the doctor's name, address and codes that are used to provide the patient with an itemized record of the services rendered.

► A Special Use

Many practices which have converted from pegboard to a computerized bookkeeping system still keep their pegboard available as a **back-up system.**

Then, should the computer be down, the pegboard can quickly be brought into use. Entries are made manually and then transferred to the computer once it is functioning again.

98

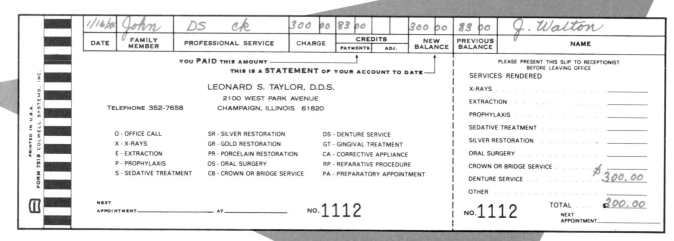

Figure 6-4. Combination receipt and charge slip used with a pegboard system.

USING THE PEGBOARD

Step #1 — Setting Up

1. Each morning place a new daily journal page on the pegboard. Date and number this sheet. If more than one page is used per day, each one is headed in a similar manner and the totals are brought forward from the previous page.

2. Place a series of receipt and charge slips into position over the journal page so that the first slip is aligned with the first blank line.

3. When a patient arrives, complete the charge slip portion of the receipt-and-charge form to show the account name and the previous balance.

4. Detach the charge slip portion along the perforation and attach it to the patient's chart to be forwarded to the treatment area.

Step #2 — Posting

1. When the completed charge slip is returned to the business office, post the charges for this visit to the patient account and to the practice records.

2. To do this, align the first blank line of the patient's ledger card with the line for the numbered charge slip.

3. Place the ledger card over the daily journal page and under the receipt form.

4. When making pegboard entries, use a ballpoint pen and press firmly so that all information will be transferred clearly.

5. Starting from the left side, enter the following information:
   * Date
   * Name of patient
   * Codes showing services rendered
   * Fees charged

6. At this point, stop and ask the patient for payment.

   If the patient makes a payment, record it.

7. Then note the new account balance.

   Remove the receipt from the pegboard and give it to the patient.

8. If using the appointment space on the receipt, write this information after the form has been removed from the pegboard.

9. If there is an outstanding balance, give the patient a return envelope with the completed receipt form and ask that payment be made as soon as possible.

▶ Step #3 — The End of the Day

1. At the end of the day, total all columns of the daily journal page (or pages for that day).

2. Complete the **proof of posting** form at the bottom of the page. (This is a double check for accuracy.)

   To do this, simply supply the totals and follow the directions on the form.

   If there is an error, it is necessary to go back and locate it immediately.

3. Complete the **cash control box** to ensure that the amount of cash and checks on hand matches the amount shown.

4. Carry the appropriate totals forward to the monthly summary sheet.

COMPUTERIZED SYSTEMS

The steps involved in using a computerized system are very similar to those for pegboard bookkeeping. Although computerized systems vary as to the specifics of how they work, the following are the basic steps to be followed throughout the day.

▶ Step #1 — Setting Up

1. At the beginning of the day, turn on the system and verify the date within the accounts receivable program. This is the date that the system will use to keep track of all posting and transactions.

2. Print, or manually prepare, charge slips for all patients scheduled to be seen that day.

▶ Step #2 — Posting

1. When the charge slip is returned to the business office, use the appropriate codes to post all charges, payments and adjustments for this patient visit.

2. Print and give to the patient a receipt or walk-out statement.

Step #3 — At the End Of The Day

1. Print the daily journal report. Double check that the entries match the information shown on the charge slips.

2. Verify that the amount of receipts shown on the system matches the amount of cash and checks in the drawer.

3. The computer will automatically carry the daily totals forward to the monthly and annual summaries.

POSTING

 Posting codes are used to speed and simplify entering transaction data into the bookkeeping system.

Codes are used to speed and simplify posting transaction data into the bookkeeping system. In a computerized system, numerical codes are used. In a manual system, letter codes are used.

Charge Codes

Charge codes are used to enter the fees for treatment provided to the patient. With a pegboard system, letter codes are used to describe the procedure and the amount is entered in the charge column. An explanation of these codes appears on the charge/receipt slip and on the bottom of the account ledger card.

In a computerized system, these codes are usually organized in a **charge code file**. Each code within this file includes the ADA procedure code number and written description of the procedure plus the fee information. When the code number is posted, the fee information is automatically entered with it.

Payment Codes

Payment codes are used to enter the description and amount of any payment received on the account. With a pegboard system, letter codes are used to describe the type or source of the payment. The amount received is entered in the payment column.

In a computerized system, these codes are usually organized in a **payment code file.** The basic payment codes are for: cash, checks and credit cards. However, further coding makes it possible to more precisely identify the source of payment.

For example, there may be codes to clarify whether the check received was a personal check (for the patient's share of the bill) or was from an insurance carrier (and to specify which carrier).

Adjustment Codes

Adjustment codes are used to change the amount of the account balance. Specific types of adjustments are discussed later in this chapter. With a pegboard system, letter codes are used to describe the reason for the adjustment.

The amount of the adjustment is entered into the adjustment column. It is assumed that adjustments are to be subtracted from the account balance. When the adjustment is to be **added** to the account balance, it is circled.

In a computerized system, these codes are usually organized in an **adjustment code file.** Each adjustment code must include instructions to the system telling it whether this adjustment acts like a payment (decreases the balance) or acts like a charge (increases the balance).

 Posting Payments

Payments By Mail

Payments received in the mail are promptly credited to the patient's account just as if the patient were present. Unless the patient requests one, it is not necessary to send a receipt for a payment by check.

When posting these payments to a pegboard system, it is not necessary to use a charge/receipt slip. Instead, the ledger card is positioned and the entry is made directly on the ledger card and through to the daily journal page.

Payment From Insurance Carriers

Generally, payments from insurance carriers will not cover the total cost of the patient's dental treatment. Therefore, the amount received from the insurance will be only partial payment and the patient is responsible for the balance.

When an insurance check comes in, it is listed in the same manner as other checks, with a notation of the name of the company paying.

For example, a payment listed as CK (BCBS) would mean a check received from Blue Cross/Blue Shield. If there is any balance due on the account, it is the patient's responsibility and should be billed accordingly.

Under certain circumstances it is not permissible to collect the balance from the patient. In this case the uncollectible balance must be written-off. This is done as an account adjustment with the amount being subtracted from the account balance.

Payments By Credit Card

Many practices honor selected credit cards as payment for dental treatment. However, before this can be done, the doctor must have signed an agreement with the credit card company.

The credit card company makes a service charge for each transaction. (This is called **discounting** and the amount is commonly in the range of 3 to 5 percent of the total amount charged.)

This fee is part of the doctor's cost of doing business and is <u>not</u> charged to the patient. The amount of the discount, or service charge, is usually handled in the checkbook as a practice expense.

When accepting a credit card payment, complete a sales agreement form and give the customer copy to the patient.

Post the transaction noting the date, name of the credit card company, and the full amount of the payment as shown on the sales slip.

▶ **Adjustments And Account Special Entries**

Examples of how these adjustments are made on a pegboard system are shown in Figure 6-5.

Discounts

Occasionally a courtesy discount will be given to a special patient or to another professional. To make such an adjustment, enter an appropriate explanation, such as *"courtesy discount,"* in the service column. A professional discount acts like a payment and is subtracted from the account balance.

Write-Offs

A write-off is that portion of the balance which cannot be collected for some reason. A write-off is an adjustment that acts like a payment and is subtracted from the account balance.

✓ With Medicaid patients, the amount of the charge which Medicaid does not pay must be written off (See Chapter 7).
✓ With some (<u>but not all</u>) insurance programs, a portion of the charge must be written off (See Chapter 7).
✓ When an account is turned over to collection, that portion of the fee which the agency keeps must be written off (See Chapter 8).

N.S.F. Checks

Also known as *returned checks,* "N.S.F." stands for **"non-sufficient funds."** When the person writing the check does not have enough money on deposit to cover the check, the bank will return it to the practice.

Usually such a check can be redeposited after a telephone call to the person who wrote it. If so, this extra transaction needs no bookkeeping entry. In redeposit, use a separate deposit slip and note on it "redeposit of (name) N.S.F. check."

If the check cannot be redeposited, the amount of the returned check must be added back to the patient's account balance.

To do this with a pegboard, position the ledger card on the daily journal page. In the services column list "N.S.F. check." Next enter the amount of the check in the adjustment column and circle the amount to indicate that it is added. Then add this amount back to the account balance.

Date	Family Member	Professional Service	Charge	Paym'ts	Adj	Balance
		Balance Forward				-0-
1/28/xx	Joyce	C+B ck	$600.00	$200.00		$400.00
1/28/xx		courtesy discount			$50.00	$350.00

A Courtesy Discount. The amount of the discount is
entered in the adjustment column and is subtracted from the balance.

Date	Family Member	Professional Service	Charge	Paym'ts	Adj	Balance
2/1/xx		Balance Forward				$80.00
2/2/xx		ck		$80.00		-0-
2/11/xx		NSF ck			($80.00)	$80.00

NSF Check. The amount of the returned check is entered
in the adjustment column and circled to indicate that this amount must be
added to the balance.

Date	Family Member	Professional Service	Charge	Paym'ts	Adj	Balance
1/2/xx		Balance Forward				$150.00
1/10/xx		refer to ABC Collection Agency				
2/11/xx		ck ABC Agency		$75.00		$75.00
2/11/xx		uncollectible balance			$75.00	-0-

Payment From A Collection Agency. The
"uncollectible balance" is entered in the adjustment column and
subtracted from the account balance.

Figure 6-5. Ledger cards showing adjustment entries.

Payments From A Collection Agency

As a fee for services, a collection agency will keep a percentage of what it collects. For accounting purposes, the amount withheld is treated as a discount.

For example, an account for $110 is turned over to an agency for collection. When the patient pays the $110 to the agency, $40 is retained by the agency and $70 is paid to the dentist.

When the $70 payment is received, it would be credited to the account. The $40 which was withheld is entered in the adjustment column and is subtracted. (This is a write-off.) This should leave the account with a zero balance.

Stop-Payment Orders

Sometimes the person writing a check will want to stop payment on that check. This may happen because the check has been lost or stolen. For example, if a check has been delayed in the mail, the patient might think it had been lost and put a stop-payment order on it.

Another reason might be a dispute over the bill which was paid with that check. Should such a dispute arise, be sure to inform the doctor of the problem immediately!

If a patient puts a stop-payment order on a check you have received, the bank will not honor the check. It is then handled like a N.S.F. check. To do this, you must add the amount of that check back to the patient's account and subtract that amount from the practice's bank account balance.

BANK DEPOSITS

All receipts should be deposited daily and the total of the deposit should equal exactly the day's receipts (Fig. 6-6). This is important because it is a vital part of the audit trail.

▶ Restrictive Check Endorsement

▶ A restrictive endorsement prevents a check from being cashed if it is stolen.

As a protective measure, checks should be rubber stamped with a restrictive endorsement, such as the one shown below, as soon as they are received (Fig. 6-7). This restrictive endorsement prevents checks from being cashed if they are stolen.

▶ Preparing The Deposit

1. Each bank deposit must be accompanied by a deposit slip which is pre-printed with the account name and number.

2. This slip should be dated and completed accurately and legibly in ink.

3. A duplicate of the deposit slip should be prepared for the practice records.

4. A single entry is noted for cash.

5. Checks are listed separately by the amount and the last name of the person writing the check.

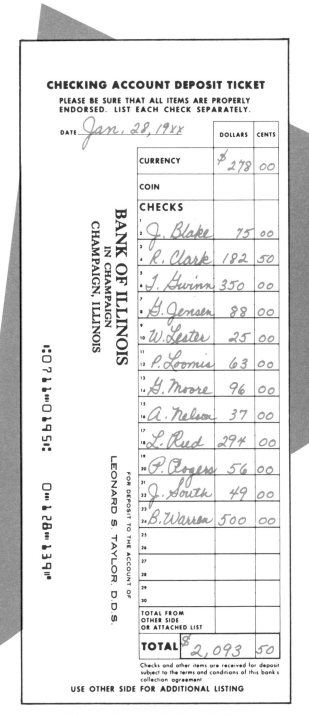

Figure 6-6. Sample deposit slip.

FOR DEPOSIT ONLY
TO THE ACCOUNT OF

Leonard S. Taylor, D.D.S.

Figure 6-7. Sample restrictive endorsement.

6. These amounts are totalled. The amount of the deposit must match the amount received for the day.

7. The date and amount of the deposit are entered in the check register. (This is discussed in Chapter 10).

Credit Card Slips

Credit card slips are <u>not</u> included with the regular daily bank deposit. Instead, they are "deposited" separately to a special bank account.

For larger volume users, the daily charges may be transmitted via telephone lines directly to the processing center. Before doing this, verify that the amounts have been accurately recorded.

Chapter

DENTAL INSURANCE

LEARNING GOALS

The student will be able to:

▶ Describe the use of a computer, and electronic claims transmission, in the management of dental insurance claims.

▶ Describe three different methods of payment for care provided under dental insurance plans.

▶ List and describe the other limitations which influence how much the carrier will pay and how much the patient must pay.

▶ Correctly use the CDT-1 procedure codes in filing claims.

▶ Complete a claim form based on information provided.

OVERVIEW OF DENTAL INSURANCE

Dental insurance is designed to increase access to dental care by reducing the cost to the patient. However, dental insurance is not designed to pay the entire cost and, in most situations, the patient remains responsible for payment of a share of the dentist's fee.

Because the patient and the insurance carrier share costs, it is necessary to see that fees are charged and collected properly from the appropriate party.

Also as a service to patients, and to facilitate claims management within the practice, it is important that all claims be completed accurately and submitted promptly.

▶ It is important that all claims be completed accurately and submitted promptly.

COMPUTERIZED CLAIMS MANAGEMENT

Using a computerized bookkeeping system greatly simplifies and speeds the preparation of insurance claims. The data necessary for producing the claim form is entered into the system as part of the account history and during posting.

✓ If the patient is to file the insurance claim, the completed claim may be printed and given to the patient before leaving the office.

✓ If the practice is to file the claim, these are usually printed and mailed at the end of the day.

▶ Electronic Claims Transmission

When a paper claim form is submitted to the carrier, the data must be entered into the carrier's computer before it can be processed and paid. This handling of paper claims increases the carrier's cost of doing business and for this reason, carriers prefer to have claims submitted electronically.

Electronic claims transmission eliminates the need for paper claim forms, delays in the mail, and the possibility for error as the claim is entered into the carrier's computer. It also speeds processing and claims can be paid much more quickly. Here is how electronic claims transmission works.

1. During the day, claim information is posted into the computer. This completes both insurance and bookkeeping records.

2. A copy of the claim may be printed for the office files.

3. At the end of the day, the claims are electronically checked for errors. For example, if a tooth number has been omitted, this error would be spotted.

4. The corrected claims are electronically prepared and transmitted by the computer via modem. (A **modem** is a telephone link between two computers.)

   Some claims may be transmitted directly to the carrier.

   Other claims are transmitted to a clearinghouse which sorts the claims and sends them (via modem) to the computer of the appropriate carrier.

5. A report indicates which claims were successfully transmitted and which the system was unable to transmit. Claims that were not transmitted for any reason, must be prepared again to be submitted with the next batch.

PATIENT INFORMATION

Patient information includes data about the family members who are entitled to receive benefits under the plan. Patient information is gathered on a patient registration form such as the one shown in Figure 1-3. This includes the patient's:

✓ Full name
✓ Sex
✓ Relationship to the insured
✓ Date of birth

This data must be complete and accurate because the claim cannot be processed without it. If information is missing or wrong, the claim will be rejected and returned for completion or correction. This means extra paperwork and a delay in receiving payment.

 ### The Insured

The insured, also known as the **subscriber,** is the person who represents the family unit in relation to the insurance plan. The subscriber is usually the employee who is earning these benefits.

 ### The Beneficiaries

A beneficiary is someone who is entitled to receive benefits under a health plan. This usually includes the insured, spouse and children. However, not all plans cover all family members. It is necessary to clarify on the patient registration form just which family members are covered and which are not.

 ### The Spouse

The spouse is the wife or husband of the insured.

The Children

For purposes of defining dependent eligibility, a **child** is a dependent who does not exceed the age as designated in the contract. Most frequently, this is age 18 years.

Coverage usually ceases when the child passes the designated age, unless the "child" is still a full-time student or is permanently handicapped.

PLAN INFORMATION

A **carrier** is an insurance company which agrees to pay benefits claimed under a dental plan. A single carrier may offer several different dental plans.

A **plan** is an insurance contract which the carrier has written to provide specific benefits to those covered by the plan.

Because insurance coverage is complex, you provide a service to the patient by helping the patient understand what benefits to expect. You will be better able to do this after you have gathered the basic plan information.

Plan information is found in the **Benefits Booklet** which is given to the subscriber. (If you don't have this plan on file, ask the patient to bring the booklet along at the first visit.)

Having plan information organized on a form such as the one shown in Figure 7-1 makes it easier to determine the patient's share of the costs.

The features, and limitations, of these plans are negotiated with the purchaser (usually an employer) of the coverage. The carrier is responsible for covering only the level of treatment included in that plan.

The method of payment and limitations within the plan are the major factors which determine how much the carrier will pay — and how much the patient must pay.

METHODS OF PAYMENT

There are many different ways in which dental plans pay for the patient's care. It is important that you understand how these different methods of payment influence the amount of payment the doctor will receive from the carrier.

Fee-For-Service

Under the fee-for-service system, the dentist is paid on the basis of services actually rendered. A major difference in these fee-for-service programs is the method by which payment is determined.

The two most commonly used methods of calculating benefits under fee-for service plans are on the basis of a Schedule of Benefits and on the basis of Usual and Customary fees.

Schedule Of Benefits

A schedule of benefits is a list of specified amounts which the carrier will pay toward the cost of covered services. Payment is based on services actually performed; however, the schedule of benefits is not related in any way to the doctor's fee schedule.

Under most schedule of benefits plans, the patient is responsible for the difference between what the carrier will pay and what the dentist actually charges. However, the amount that the patient actually pays will also be influenced by the other factors in the patient's plan.

Usual and Customary

Usual and customary payment is based on the doctor's fee schedule as it relates to that of other dentists in the area.

In this situation, **usual fee** means the fee that is usually charged, for a given service, by a dentist to private patients. These fees are determined by the individual doctor and are reflected in the carrier's records as that dentist's **fee profile.**

DENTAL INSURANCE PLAN SUMMARY FORM

PLAN NAME __Ace Automotive__
PLAN/GROUP NUMBER __AA 1242__

CARRIER NAME __Continental Insurance Company__
CARRIER ADDRESS __555 E. Wacker Drive, Chicago, IL 60612__
CONTACT PERSON __Alice Gibbons__
TELEPHONE NUMBER __312-471-0821__

EMPLOYER NAME __Ace Automotive__
EMPLOYER ADDRESS __Urbana, IL__
CONTACT PERSON __Mr. Lester Norton__
TELEPHONE NUMBER __351-2014__

PAYMENT: UCR _____ SCHEDULE OF BENEFITS __XX__
(If available, file copy of schedule behind this page.)

ACCEPT ASSIGNMENT: YES _____ NO __XX__
PRE-TREATMENT ESTIMATE REQUIRED: YES __XX__ NO _____
ALTERNATIVE PROCEDURE POLICY: YES __XX__ NO _____

CO-INSURANCE:
　　Preventive __100__
　　Routine __70__
　　Major __50__

DEDUCTIBLE: __$50__
(Indicate: (annual) or lifetime, (individual) or family.)

EXCLUSIONS: _____
EXCLUSIONS: _____

MAXIMUM: Annual _____
MAXIMUM: Lifetime _____

OTHER: _____

Figure 7-1. Insurance plan summary form.

The **customary fee** for a given service is set by the carrier. The carrier sets the customary fee at a percentile of the usual fees charged by dentists with similar training and experience within the same geographic area. The Table *"Understanding The 90th Percentile"* explains how this concept is applied.

 HMO

A **health maintenance organization** (HMO) is a health care delivery system in which the patient pays a flat monthly premium to the HMO (this may be paid through the patient's employer). The premium covers all dental services as specified in the contract.

The patient must select a dentist from a list of providers either employed by the HMO, or under contract to the HMO.

- Under a **capitation plan**, the dentists are paid a flat fee for each patient under the practice's care, regardless of the amount of care provided.
- Under a **noncapitation plan**, the dentists are paid according to the number of patients seen, or amount of treatment provided, over a given period of time.
- Under either type of plan, the patient may be required to make a co-payment for each visit.

 PPO

A **preferred provider organization** (PPO) is a formal agreement to treat a specific patient population (such as the members of a large union) at an agreed upon rate.

This rate is usually a discounted fee-for-service. Because the discount is offered, the providers are designated "preferred providers" by the organizing group.

Patients may select their own dentist; however, they have the incentive to select the "preferred providers" because a larger portion of the costs will be covered under this arrangement.

IPA

An **independent practice association** (IPA) is a type of HMO. IPA's are generally formed and run by dentists who enter into agreements with organizations (usually employers) to provide dental services to a defined group of persons (usually employees).

IPA dentists usually practice out of their own offices. Many continue to see their regular patients on a fee-for-service basis, while seeing IPA patients at the IPA rate.

UNDERSTANDING THE 90th PERCENTILE	
When the customary fee is set at the 90th percentile, it means that this fee, or a lesser amount, is charged for this service by 9 out of 10 doctors in that area.	For example, in Dr. Taylor's community 9 out of 10 doctors charge $40 for service XYZ.
If the doctor's usual fee is <u>exactly the same</u> as the customary fee, the physician will be paid the actual amount of his or her usual fee.	If Dr. Taylor charges $40 for XYZ service, his fee will be paid in full. He will receive $40 because $40 is his usual fee.
If the doctor's usual fee is <u>less than</u> the customary fee, the physician will be paid the actual amount of his or her usual fee.	If Dr. Taylor charges $35 for XYZ service, his fee will be paid in full. He will receive $35 (not $40) because $35 is his usual fee.
If the doctor's usual fee is <u>more than</u> the customary fee, the physician will be paid only the amount of the customary fee.	If Dr. Taylor charges $45 for XYZ service, his fee will <u>not</u> be paid in full. He will receive $40 (not $45) because $40 is the customary fee for this service.

GOVERNMENT PROGRAMS

▶ Medicaid

Medicaid is a government program to provide health and dental care for the poor. This program is governed by rules set forth in each state. Therefore, coverage and eligibility vary from state to state. In some states, the patient may be responsible for a small coinsurance payment at each visit.

Payment is based on a schedule of benefits and the dentist must accept the amount paid by the carrier as payment in full. This means that the doctor <u>may not</u> bill the patient for the difference between the usual fee and the amount that Medicaid has paid.

▶ Medicare

There is no coverage under Medicare for routine dental care.

LIMITATIONS

The following factors influence the amount of benefits the beneficiary is entitled to receive under a plan, and how much is the beneficiary's share of these costs.

▶ Eligibility

The first factor to consider is to be certain that the patient is eligible to receive benefits under this plan. If in doubt, contact the carrier and determine eligibility before the patient owes a large balance.

▶ If in doubt about the patient's eligibility, contact the carrier before the patient owes a large balance.

▶ Deductible

The deductible is the stipulated amount that the covered person must pay toward the cost of covered dental treatment before the benefits of the program go into effect.

This may be an individual or a family deductible. For example:

- The plan covering George Adams and his family has an individual deductible of $150 per year. Each year that amount of covered dental expenses must be paid for each family member before that family member is eligible for plan benefits.
- The plan covering the Hubbard family has a family deductible of $500 per year. Each year total covered dental expenses for family members must reach $500 before the plan benefits become effective.

► Coinsurance

Coinsurance, also known as **copayment,** is a provision of a program by which the beneficiary shares in the cost of covered expenses on a percentage basis.

As shown in the Table *"Coinsurance Variables,"* the amount that the patient is responsible for varies according to the policy.

Coinsurance percentages are usually listed showing the portion which the carrier will pay. To calculate the patient's share subtract this from 100%. For example, the following are commonly used co-insurance percentages.

- 100% for **preventive services** such as a recall prophy and exam. (The patient does not have any coinsurance responsibility here.)
- 70% for **routine services** such as restorations. (The patient must pay 30%.)
- 50% for **major services** such as dentures or partials. (The patient must pay 50%.)

COINSURANCE VARIABLES	
Henry Jones has a policy which pays on a Usual and Customary basis.	Martha Jackson has a policy which pays on a schedule of benefits.
The fee is $200 for restorative services.	The fee is $200 for restorative services.
Henry's policy fully covers the doctor's fee.	Martha's carrier allows $180 for this service.
	Martha is responsible for the $20 difference between the doctor's fee and the carrier's schedule of benefits basis.
The co-insurance is 70%.	The co-insurance is 70%.
The carrier will pay $140 (which is 70% of $200).	The carrier will pay $126 (which is 70% of $180).
Henry is responsible for $60 (which is 30% of $200).	Martha is responsible for $54 (which is 30% of $180).
Henry must pay a total of $60.	Martha must pay a total of $74.

Exclusions

Some policies exclude certain services such as cosmetic dentistry. This means that the carrier will not pay for this service. The patient may still receive the treatment; however, the patient is responsible for the entire fee.

Maximums

The carrier may establish a maximum as to the amount that will be paid for dental benefits within a given year, or for a lifetime.

For example, a plan may have a $1,000 **annual maximum** per patient per year. This means that the carrier will not pay for any treatment beyond that amount even if the treatment is a "covered service."

The plan may also include a **lifetime maximum** of $2,000 for orthodontic treatment. This means that the carrier will not pay more than this amount in orthodontic benefits for this patient no matter how long the treatment takes.

Alternative Benefit Policy

When there is more than one treatment option available, under an alternative benefit policy, the carrier reserves the right to pay only for the less expensive treatment.

For example, the patient has a missing tooth which may be replaced with a fixed bridge (for $2,500) or with a removable partial denture (for $750). In this situation, the carrier has the right to pay benefits only for the partial denture.

The patient may have the bridge placed; however, the carrier will pay benefits only as if the partial had been made. The patient is responsible for the difference in the fee.

An alternative benefit policy is not a statement by the carrier that one form of treatment is better than another. It is simply a way of controlling costs.

Coordination Of Benefits (COB)

When a patient has insurance coverage under more than one group plan, this is known as **dual coverage** and it is necessary to coordinate the benefits.

Under coordination of benefits, the patient may not receive payment from both carriers that comes to <u>more than</u> 100% of the actual dental expenses.

In order to coordinate benefits, it is necessary to determine which carrier is **primary** (and should pay first) and which carrier is **secondary** (and should pay at least a portion of the balance).

✓ The primary carrier is listed at the top right of the claim form.
✓ The secondary carrier information is listed in answer to questions 11-15 on the claim form.

Many carriers have automatic coordination of benefits, and the primary carrier will forward the claim to the secondary carrier for payment of benefits. If there is not automatic coordination of benefits:

1. Submit the claim first to the primary carrier.

2. When payment is received, it will be accompanied by an **explanation of benefits** (EOB).

    Send the claim, along with a copy of the EOB, to the secondary carrier.

Determining The Primary And Secondary Carrier

When the patient is also the insured, the patient's carrier is primary and the spouse's carrier is secondary.

*   When *Mrs. Smith* comes in as a patient, her carrier is primary.
    Mr. Smith's carrier is secondary.
*   When *Mr. Smith* comes in as a patient, his carrier is primary.
    Mrs. Smith's carrier is secondary.

The Birthday Rule

▶ For children with dual coverage, the primary carrier is determined by the birthday rule.

When the *Smith children* come in, it is a different situation. For children with dual coverage, the primary carrier is usually determined by the birthday rule.

The carrier for the parent who has a birthday earlier in the year is primary. This has nothing to do with which parent is older.

For example, if *Mrs. Smith's* birthday is in <u>January</u> and *Mr. Smith's* birthday is in <u>July</u>, *Mrs. Smith's* carrier is primary in providing coverage for the Smith children.

▶ Pre-Treatment Estimate

Knowing how much the carrier will pay is very helpful in making financial arrangements for the patient's share of the costs. One way to get this information is to submit the treatment plan to the carrier for a pre-treatment estimate. (This is also known as **predetermination.**) The response from the carrier should include information regarding:

*   The patient's eligibility.
*   Covered services and benefit amounts payable.
*   Application of appropriate deductibles, coinsurance and/or maximum limitations.

In some situations, such as when the cost of planned treatment exceeds $500, the carrier may require that a pre-treatment estimate be submitted so that treatment can be authorized. If this is a requirement of the plan and it is not done, the carrier may deny benefits to the patient.

When submitting a pre-treatment estimate, check the appropriate box at the top left of the claim form. Where the claim asks for "*Date Service Performed,*" leave this space blank. (These are planned services, not treatment that has already been provided.)

The carrier may ask that radiographs be submitted with the request for the pre-treatment estimate. If a dual film packet was used when the x-rays were taken, the "extra set" of films is sent. If these are not available, the original films are duplicated and the duplicates are submitted to the carrier. Under no circumstances are the original films submitted.

CDT-1 PROCEDURE CODES

For insurance reporting purposes, it is necessary to use codes to describe the dental services provided to the patients. The CDT-1 procedure codes, published by the American Dental Association, are used for this purpose.

▶ A CDT-1 code is used to describe the procedure.

▶ How CDT-1 Codes Work

As shown in the Table "*CDT-1 Categories Of Services,*" The CDT codes are divided into twelve categories. Each category includes a range of code numbers. These codes share the following characteristics:

- Each procedure code has five numerals.
- The first number is always 0, which indicates that this concerns a dental procedure.
- The second number indicates the category of dental service. For example, "03" is an endodontic service.
- The remaining numbers indicate specific services within each group. (When coding, always select the code which exactly describes the procedure which was performed.)
- A number ending in 999 indicates an unspecified code which is used to identify a procedure not fully explained in that coding group. For example, 04999 is the unspecified code for periodontics.
  When a 999 code is used, the claim must be accompanied by a written narrative report which fully describes the procedure.

The Table "*CDT-1 Code Samples*" shows examples of these codes. Each code is very specific. You must pay very close attention to every word in the description and select the correct code! Use of the wrong code may result in lower benefits, or in having benefits denied altogether. The following are examples of specifics to look for:

- **Oral examinations** — There are separate codes for initial, periodic (recall), and emergency examinations.
- **Restorations** — Each code is specific as to the type of restorative material and the tooth surfaces restored.
  A **resin restoration** is commonly referred to as a *composite restoration.*
  A **single crown,** is coded as a restoration.
- **Fixed Prosthodontics** — Each unit (pontic or retainer) of a **bridge,** is coded separately. (A retainer is also known as an *abutment.*)

CDT-1 CATEGORIES OF SERVICES		
Category	**Service**	**Code Series**
I.	Diagnostic	00100-00999
II.	Preventive	01000-01999
III.	Restorative	02000-02999
IV.	Endodontics	03000-03999
V.	Periodontics	04000-04999
VI.	Prosthodontics, removable	05000-05899
VII.	Maxillofacial Prosthetics	05900-05999
VIII.	Implant Services	06000-06199
IX.	Prosthodontics, fixed	06200-06999
X.	Oral Surgery	07000-07999
XI.	Orthodontics	08000-08999
XII.	Adjunctive General Services	09000-09999

▶ The Noble Metal Classification System

The metals used in cast restorations are alloys. (An **alloy** is a mixture of two or more metals.) For coding purposes, the noble metal classification system is used to identify these alloys.

The **noble metals** are *gold* (Au), *palladium* (Pd), and *platinum* (Pt). All other metals are considered to be **base metals**. For coding purposes, the alloy is described by the proportion of noble metals it contains. The three groups of alloys are:

✓ High noble.
✓ Noble.
✓ Predominantly base.

The codes for cast restorations are specific as to the type of alloy that was used. Information regarding the type of alloy used may be obtained from the dentist, or by referring to the written laboratory prescription.

THE CLAIM FORM

A dental insurance claim form is used to submit a treatment plan for a pre-treatment estimate and to request payment of claims for services that have been rendered.

The *Dental Claim Form,* as shown in Figure 7-2, is accepted by most dental insurance carriers.

The claim form has three primary information areas. Patient and subscriber information is at the top, provider identification information is in the middle, and the balance of the form is used for treatment information.

| CDT-1 CODE SAMPLES ||
Code #	Procedure Description
00110	Initial oral examination
00120	Periodic oral examination
00210	Radiographs — Intraoral-complete series (including bitewings)
00220	Radiographs — Intraoral-periapical-first film
00230	Radiographs — Intraoral-periapical-each additional film
00272	Radiographs — Bitewings, two films
00330	Radiographs — Panoramic film
01110	Prophylaxis-adult
01120	Prophylaxis-child
01201	Topical application of fluoride (including prophylaxis)-child
01203	Topical application of fluoride (excluding prophylaxis)-child
02110	Amalgam, one-surface, primary
02120	Amalgam, two-surface, primary
02140	Amalgam, one-surface, permanent
02150	Amalgam, two-surface, permanent
02330	Resin-one surface, anterior
02331	Resin-two surfaces, anterior
02790	Crown-full cast high noble metal
05110	Complete denture, upper
05120	Complete denture, lower
06210	Pontic-cast high noble metal
06790	Crown-full cast high noble metal
07110	Extraction, single tooth
07120	Extraction, each additional tooth

▶ Check One

In the upper left corner of the claim form, check the appropriate box to indicate:

☐ Dentist's pre-treatment estimate.

☐ Dentist's statement of actual services.

▶ Carrier Name And Address

Enter the carrier name and address in the box at the upper right corner of the claim form.

Dental Claim Form

Check one:

☐ Dentist's pre-treatment estimate

☐ Dentist's statement of actual services

Carrier name and address

DELTA DENTAL OF ILLINOIS
500 STATE PLAZA
SPRINGFIELD, ILLINOIS

PATIENT COVERAGE INFORMATION

1. Patient name first / m.i. / last	2. Relationship to employee	3. Sex m f	4. Patient birthdate MM DD YYYY	5. If full time student school city
GERALDINE WILLIAMS	☒ self ☐ child ☐ spouse ☐ other____	x	04 25 50	

6. Employee/subscriber name and mailing address	7. Employee/subscriber soc. sec. or I.D. number	8. Employee/subscriber birthdate MM DD YYYY	9. Employer (company) name and address	10. Group number
P.O. BOX 215 CENTERVILLE, IL 61822	543-20-9765	04 25 50	FIRST BANK OF CENTERVILLE	FBOC-333-45

11. Is patient covered by another dental plan? yes ☒ no If yes, complete 12-a.
Is patient covered by a medical plan? yes ☒ no

12-a. Name and address of carrier(s)

12-b. Group no.(s)

13. Name and address of other employer(s)

14-a. Employee/subscriber name (if different than patient's)	14-b. Employee/subscriber soc. sec. or I.D. number	14-c. Employee/subscriber birthdate MM DD YYYY	15. Relationship to patient ☐ self ☐ parent ☐ spouse ☐ other____

I have reviewed the following treatment plan. I authorize release of any information relating to this claim. I understand that I am responsible for all costs of dental treatment.

▶ SIGNATURE ON FILE   2/1/XX

Signed (Patient, or parent if minor)   Date

I hereby authorize payment of the dental benefits otherwise payable to me directly to the below named dental entity.

▶ SIGNATURE ON FILE   2/1/XX

Signed (Insured person)   Date

BILLING DENTIST

16. Name of Billing Dentist or Dental Entity
LEONARD S. TAYLOR, D.D.S.

17. Address where payment should be remitted
2100 WEST PARK AVENUE

City, State, Zip
CHAMPAIGN, IL 61820

18. Dentist Soc. Sec. or T.I.N.	19. Dentist license no.	20. Dentist phone no.
123-45-6789	12345	351-5400

21. First visit date current series	22. Place of treatment Office Hosp. ECF Other	23. Radiographs or models enclosed? No ☒ Yes How many?
2/1/XX		

	No	Yes	If yes, enter brief description and dates
24. Is treatment result of occupational illness or injury?	X		
25. Is treatment result of auto accident?	X		
26. Other accident?	X		
27. If prosthesis, is this initial placement?	X		(If no, reason for replacement)
29. Is treatment for orthodontics?	X		

28. Date of prior placement

If services already commenced enter: Date appliances placed Mos. treatment remaining

---

Identify missing teeth with "x"

FACIAL — UPPER RIGHT / LEFT — LINGUAL — PRIMARY / PERMANENT — LOWER — FACIAL

Tooth # or letter	Surface	Description of service (including x-rays, prophylaxis, materials used, etc.)	Date service performed Mo. Day Year	Procedure number	Fee	For administrative use only
		INITIAL ORAL EXAMINATION	2 1 XX 0	0110	25 00	
		INTRAORAL-COMPLETE SERIES	2 1 XX 0	0210	50 00	
		DIAGNOSTIC CASTS	2 1 XX 0	0470	25 00	
		PROPHYLAXIS-ADULT	2 1 XX 0	1110	35 00	
	MOD	SEDATIVE FILLING	2 1 XX 0	2940	15 00	

31. Remarks for unusual services

I hereby certify that the procedures as indicated by date have been completed and that the fees submitted are the actual fees I have charged and intend to collect for those procedures.

▶

Signed (Treating Dentist)   License Number   Date

Total Fee Charged	$150 00
Max. Allowable	
Deductible	
Carrier %	
Carrier pays	
Patient pays	

Figure 7-2. Insurance claim form sample.

▶ Patient Information

Questions 1 through 10 ask for information regarding the patient and the primary carrier. Questions 11 through 15 ask for information regarding secondary coverage.

▶ Assignment Of Benefits

Assignment of benefits is a procedure whereby the subscriber authorizes the carrier to make payment of allowable benefits directly to the dentist. If there is no assignment of benefits, the check will go directly to the patient.

To assign the benefits, the subscriber signs the appropriate box on the insurance claim form. When benefits have been assigned, the carrier is responsible for sending the check directly to the dentist.

If benefits have been assigned, financial arrangements are usually made only for the patient's share of the cost.

If there is no assignment of benefits, financial arrangements are made for the total amount of the fee — just as if the patient did not have dental insurance.

▶ Release Of Information

Information regarding the patient's treatment is confidential and may be released only with the patient's written consent.

A "Release of Information" box is located on the claim form next to the "Assignment of Benefits" box. The patient's signature here gives the dentist permission to reveal information regarding dental treatment to the insurance carrier.

▶ Signature On File

Having the patient's signature on file, makes it possible to complete and submit the claim even when the patient is not available to sign the completed claim form.

Also, having the patient's signature on file is essential when submitting claims electronically, because in this situation there is no "paper claim" form to be signed.

A patient registration form, such as the one shown in Figure 1-3, includes signature boxes very similar to those on the claim form. When completing the registration form, the patient should sign and date these signature boxes.

These signatures must be updated periodically. In some instances, the frequency of the update depends upon the carrier. In other situations, the frequency of the update depends upon state law.

▶ Billing Dentist

Questions 16 through 20 request information to identify the dentist who has supplied these services.

▶ Background Information

Questions 21 through 29 request important background information regarding the patient's treatment.

▶ Examination And Treatment Plan

Question 30 is where you list the services provided (or planned services if this is a pre-treatment estimate).

- Use the Universal Numbering System.
- Include the tooth number, or letter, and surfaces when necessary.
- Complete the written description of the procedure.
- If this is a request for payment, enter the date of service.
- If this is a pre-treatment estimate, do not enter the date of service.
- Enter the proper procedure code number.
- Enter the total fee. (Do not subtract any portion of the fee which the patient has paid.)

▶ Remarks For Unusual Services

This space may be used to enter a brief narrative report. If a longer report is required, it should be submitted on a separate page that is clearly labeled with identification information for both the dentist and patient.

THE SUPERBILL

A superbill is a single or multi-part form that is used to simplify reporting treatment information. As shown in Figure 7-3, a superbill contains practice identification information, plus space to record treatment and fee information.

Superbills may be used with either manual or computerized bookkeeping systems. On a pegboard system, a superbill is often used in place of a receipt and charge slip.

The treatment portion of the superbill is completed in the treatment area at the end of the patient's visit. The appropriate procedure codes are circled to indicate what services were provided, and the appropriate fees are entered.

If a procedure that is not listed on the superbill was performed, it is necessary to write in the correct code, description and fee. (Remember, accuracy in coding is always important.)

In the business office, the bookkeeping entries are completed. If a multi-part superbill is used, the parts are separated.

✓ One copy stays in the office as part of the practice records.
✓ Another copy is given to the patient as a receipt for the day's visit.

Some carriers will accept a claim with a copy of the superbill taped in place over the treatment area portion of the claim form. Other carriers will not accept claims prepared in this manner. (It is best to check with the carrier prior to submitting a claim with a superbill attached.)

PEGBOARD ENTRIES

PROCEDURE CODES

DATE	FAMILY MEMBER	PROFESSIONAL SERVICE	CHARGE	CREDITS		NEW BALANCE	PREVIOUS BALANCE	NAME
				PAYMENTS	ADJ.			
2/2/	Pat	EX, P	57 00	50 00		78 00	71 00	J. Douglass

YOU **PAID** THIS AMOUNT
THIS IS A **STATEMENT** OF YOUR ACCOUNT TO DATE

Date of Service _____

Patient's Name _____

ATTENDING DENTIST'S STATEMENT | **UNIVERSAL TOOTH NUMBERING SYSTEM**

I. DIAGNOSTIC   FEE 22.00
00110   Initial Oral Examination
00120   Periodic Oral Examination
00130   Emergency Oral Examination
00210   Intraoral - Complete Series (Including Bitewings)
00220   Intraoral Periapical - Single, First Film
00230   Intraoral Periapical - Each Additional Film
00270   Bitewing Single
00272   Bitewings - Two Films
00460   Pulp Vitality Tests
00470   Diagnostic Casts

II. PREVENTIVE   35.00
01110   Adults Prophylaxis
01120   Children Prophylaxis
01210   Topical Application of Fluoride - One Treatment (Excluding Prophylaxis)
01330   Oral Hygiene Instruction
01350   Topical Application of Sealants - Per Tooth: Teeth

III. SPACE MANAGEMENT THERAPY
01510   Fixed - Unilateral Type
01515   Fixed - Bilateral Type
01520   Removable - Unilateral Type
01525   Removable - Bilateral Type

IV. ENDODONTICS
03110   Pulp Cap Direct (Excluding Final Restoration)
03120   Pulp Cap Indirect (Excluding Final Restoration)
03220   Vital Pulpotomy
03310   Root Canal Therapy - 1 Canal
03320   Root Canal Therapy - 2 Canals
03330   Root Canal Therapy - 3 Canals
03950   Canal Prep and Fitting of Preformed Dowel or Post
03960   Bleaching of Non Vital Discolored Tooth

V. PERIODONTICS
04120   Gingival Curettage Per Quadrant _____ Quadrants
04341   Scale & Root Plane Per Quad. _____ Sextants
04210   Gingivectomy Per Quadrant _____ Quadrants
04211   Gingivectomy Per Sextant _____ Sextants
04320   Provisional Splinting - Intracoronal
04330   Occlusal Adjustment (Limited)
04331   Occlusal Adjustment (Complete)
04910   Periodontal Prophylaxis

RETURN: _____ Days _____ Weeks _____ Months

VI. RESTORATIVE
02100 Amalgam Restorations

CODE	TOOTH	SURFACE	FEE
021			
021			
021			
021			
021			
021			

02300 Composite Restorations

023			
023			
023			
023			
023			
023			

02700-02899 Crowns-Single-Restorations Only

027			
027			
027			
027			
028			
028			
028			
028			

VII. PROSTHODONTICS, FIXED
06200 Bridge Pontics

062		
062		
062		
062		

06700 Crowns

067		
067		
067		
067		
067		

Other Restorative Services

	TOOTH	FEE
02920 Recement Crowns		
02940 Fillings (Sedative)		
02950 Crown Buildups - Pin Related		

Other _____

NEXT APPT.   Mon Feb. 20   1   AM PM

DAY   MONTH   DATE   TIME

VIII. PROSTHODONTICS, REMOVABLE
   Complete Dentures
05110   Complete Upper
05120   Complete Lower
05130   Immediate Upper
05140   Immediate Lower
   Partial Dentures
05241   Lower - With Chrome Lingual Bar and Two Clasps Cast Base
05261   Upper- With Chrome Palatal Bar and Two Clasps Cast Base
05310   Each Additional Clasp with Rest

054___ Adjustment to Denture
056___ Repairs to Denture
057___ Reline to Denture
05850   Tissue Conditioning
06930   Recement Bridge

IX. ORAL SURGERY   TOOTH
07110   Single Tooth Extraction
07120   Each Additional Tooth
07210   Surgical Extraction of Tooth - Erupted
07250   Root Recovery (Surgical Removal of Residual Root)
07970   Excision of Hyperplastic Tissue

X. ORTHODONTICS
   Minor Treatment for Tooth Guidance
08110   Space Maintainer Removable
08120   Space Maintainer Fixed

XI. ADJUNCTIVE GENERAL SERVICES
09110   Palliative (Emergency) Treatment of Dental Pain, Minor Procedures
09200   Anesthesia Local
09230   Analgesia
09910   Application of Desensitizing Medicaments

☐ This is a pre-treatment estimate - Circled fees are for services performed:

Today's   Treatment
Charges $_____   Estimate $_____

Notice to Insurance Carriers: This form has been adopted to keep paperwork costs down. If your own form or itemized bill is required, it will be completed upon the receipt of $10.00.

Dentist's Signature _____ D.D.S.

LEONARD S. TAYLOR, D.D.S.
2100 WEST PARK AVENUE
CHAMPAIGN, ILLINOIS 61820
Telephone (217) 351-5400

IRS # 00-1234567
S.S. # 000-00-0000

No. 1001

FORM 7567 COLWELL CO · CHAMPAIGN, ILLINOIS

TREATMENT INFORMATION

DENTIST IDENTIFICATION INFORMATION

NEXT APPOINTMENT

Figure 7-3. Superbill sample.

When submitting a claim with a superbill attachment, it is necessary to complete all other portions of the claim form. Then the superbill is taped securely in place. Staples are <u>not</u> used.

STEPS IN COMPLETING CLAIMS

 ### Before The Patient's First Visit

When the patient calls for an appointment, ask about dental insurance. If the patient has insurance coverage, request that the patient bring the identification card and benefits booklet along to the first visit.

 ### At The Patient's First Visit

Ask the patient to complete a registration form and examine the subscriber's identification card to verify coverage.

You may want to make a photocopy of this card for your records just in case you need to double check any of this information. Be sure to return the original card to the patient.

The patient should be informed of any deductible, co-insurance, or benefit limitations for which the patient is financially responsible. Definite financial arrangements should be made for payment of the patient's share.

 ### At The End Of The Patient's Visit

All charges are entered into the patient's account history (just as if the patient did not have insurance). In most practices, the patient is billed until payment is received from both carrier and patient.

For most treatment, the claim can be filed at the time of the visit. However, some procedures such as dentures or crown and bridge which require several visits, are handled differently.

For these procedures, the full amount of the fee is charged to the patient's account at the time of the visit when the procedure is started. For example, when the preparation is cut for a crown or when the preliminary impression is taken for a denture.

Although the patient's account is charged at this time, the carrier will not pay the claim until the treatment has been completed. That is, when the denture is placed or the crown is cemented.

File The Claim

All claims must be neat, complete and easy to read. If you are using a computerized bookkeeping system, it will prepare the claim for you. If you are using a manual bookkeeping system, type the claim or print it very neatly in ink.

Claims should be completed in duplicate, or photocopied, so that one copy goes to the carrier and the other stays in the office as part of the practice records.

First, complete all of the patient information portion. This data should be available on the patient registration form.

The claim form should be preprinted with the practice identification information. If it is not, enter that information.

The next step is to complete the treatment information portion.

- Answer all questions.
- Select the correct CDT-1 code to describe the patient's treatment.
- Enter appropriate fee for each service rendered.

▶ Follow-Up On Claims

Unpaid insurance claims represent money owed to the practice, and it is necessary to follow up on them.

Never file the claim form in the patient's chart. Instead, maintain a separate file for unpaid claims. Once the claim has been paid it should be removed from this file.

Follow the doctor's instructions as to whether these claim forms are maintained in a separate "paid" file, or are discarded.

If a claim is not paid within 30 days, contact the carrier to determine if there is a problem.

If a carrier returns a claim because of an error or missing information, make the necessary corrections and re-submit the claim as quickly as possible.

Chapter

COLLECTIONS
AND
PAYMENT PLANS

LEARNING GOALS

The student will be able to:

▶ Describe the following payment plans: payment at the time of treatment, statements, divided payments and office budget plan.

▶ State the conditions under which a Truth in Lending form is required.

▶ Demonstrate the use of an estimate sheet in making financial arrangements.

▶ Describe the use of an accounts receivable report and state how to calculate the age of an account.

▶ Demonstrate making collection calls.

▶ Describe the use of collection agencies to collect overdue accounts.

▶ Describe the use of small claims court to collect overdue accounts.

OVERVIEW OF COLLECTIONS AND PAYMENT PLANS

If the dentist is to be able to continue providing quality care for patients, he or she must maintain a financially successful practice. In order to do this, the dentist charges a fair fee for professional services provided. These **fees charged** represent the dentist's *potential earnings*.

The **payments** received from the collection of these fees make up the dentist's *actual income*. And, it is only from this actual income that practice overhead costs, including staff salaries, can be paid.

A financially successful practice is operated in a business-like manner. This includes having clearly stated policies regarding the:

✓ Payment plans to be offered to patients.
✓ Procedures for making financial arrangements.
✓ Routine steps for collecting overdue accounts.

PAYMENT PLANS

In an effort to help patients finance their dental care, the dentist will usually offer a choice of payment plans. Those most commonly available are: payment at the time of treatment, monthly statements, divided payments and office budget plans.

Payment At The Time Of Treatment

This is also known as being on a **cash basis.** This policy requires that all fees be paid in full at the time of each visit (Fig. 8-1). Payment may be made in cash, by check or with a credit card.

This payment plan helps to control practice costs, reduce the number of statements to be mailed each month, improve cash flow and minimize collection problems. It also creates a financial problem for some patients.

▶ Overdue accounts require prompt follow-up.

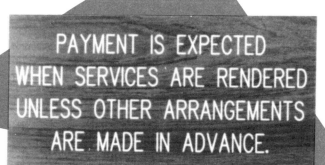

PAYMENT IS EXPECTED WHEN SERVICES ARE RENDERED UNLESS OTHER ARRANGEMENTS ARE MADE IN ADVANCE.

Figure 8-1. Sign which may be used to inform patients that payment is expected at the time of treatment.

Implementing A Cash Policy

- Notify the patient of this policy <u>before</u> the appointment. If possible, give an estimate as to how much the fees will be for this visit.
- Do not be timid about asking for payment. At the end of the visit state, *"Mr. Jones the fee for today's visit is $75. Will you be taking care of that with cash, check or credit card?"*
- If the patient is not prepared to pay, and has insurance, try to collect at least the patient's share of the cost.
- If a patient fails to make a payment, give a walk-out statement with a reply envelope, and ask that payment be mailed as soon as possible.

Offering Cash Discounts

Because the practice saves overhead expenses when it is not necessary to track and collect money owed, some practices offer the patient a small discount (usually 5% or less) in exchange for payment, in full, in advance.

A patient receives a cash discount when the entire amount of the treatment plan is paid in advance. To handle this for bookkeeping purposes, as treatment is provided, the fee for each service is posted in full, and the amount of the discount is subtracted as an account adjustment.

▶ **Monthly Statements**

Statements are due when received — and should be paid <u>in full</u> within 30 days. For this reason, statements are considered to be a **modified-cash** policy. A reply envelope is included with the statement to encourage prompt payment.

It is important that statements are mailed on time each month on a 30-day cycle. This helps patients handle their obligations in a business-like manner. It also helps to assure a steady cash flow for the practice.

Itemized Statements

The more information that is included on the statement (and the more easily the patient can understand the statement), the more likely the patient is to pay it. Therefore, the statement should be itemized to show at least these details:

- The date of each visit during the billing cycle.
- The name of the patient treated during each of these visits.
- The services provided and fees charged at each visit.
- All payments and credits received on the account.
- The current balance for the account.

Manual System Statements

With a pegboard system, the account ledger card is usually photocopied to provide a detailed and accurate statement (Fig. 8-2). The ledger entries should be legible, and the photocopy should be of good quality so that the resulting statement will be professional in appearance.

STATEMENT

LEONARD S. TAYLOR, D.D.S.
2100 WEST PARK AVENUE
CHAMPAIGN, ILLINOIS 61822

TELEPHONE 367-6671

Mr. James A. Gridley
670 Northridge Terrace
Champaign, IL 61820

DATE	FAMILY MEMBER	PROFESSIONAL SERVICE	CHARGE	CREDITS PAYM'TS	CREDITS ADJ	BALANCE
1/2/xx		BALANCE FORWARD				$25.00
1/9/xx	James	SR S2	$45 00	$25 00		45 00
1/15/xx	Ruth	GT	125 00			170 00
2/10/xx		ck		170 00		– 0 –
2/15/xx	Ruth	C + B	400 00			400 00
2/18/xx	Jimmy	FT	18 00			418 00

1625

PAY LAST AMOUNT IN THIS COLUMN ⌂

O - OFFICE CALL	SR - SILVER RESTORATION	DS - DENTURE SERVICE
X - X-RAYS	GR - GOLD RESTORATION	GT - GINGIVAL TREATMENT
E - EXTRACTION	PR - PORCELAIN RESTORATION	CA - CORRECTIVE APPLIANCE
P - PROPHYLAXIS	OS - ORAL SURGERY	RP - REPARATIVE PROCEDURE
S - SEDATIVE TREATMENT	CB - CROWN OR BRIDGE SERVICE	PA - PREPARATORY APPOINTMENT

Figure 8-2. Photocopied pegboard statement sample.

After the ledger cards have been photocopied, each resulting statement must be folded and placed in a window envelope along with a reply envelope. The window envelope is then sealed and a postage stamp is added.

Typewritten statements are another alternative. These statements are usually **semi-itemized.** This means that they contain some detail, such as the name and charges for each family member for the month, but not as much detail as an itemized statement.

Computer Generated Statements

A computerized accounts receivable system easily generates itemized statements. When a "mailer" is used (in which the statement and envelope is combined in one form), there is little additional mailing preparation to be done after the statements are printed.

When continuous feed statement forms are used, the computer prints the statements. Then the forms must be separated and prepared for mailing. These are the same steps that must be carried out for photocopied statements.

Cycle Billing

Most practices mail statements at the end of the month. However, cycle billing is used if there are too many statements to be handled at one time during the month.

In cycle billing, statements for the first half of the alphabet may be mailed before the 15th of the month and the second half can be mailed at the end of the month.

If the job is still too large, cycle billing can be further divided so that some patients are billed each week, or daily, if necessary. However, instead of increasing the frequency of billing, it is better to improve collections and thereby reduce the number of statements being sent.

Finance Charges

Some dentists make a finance charge on all overdue balances. If this is the practice policy, the patient should be informed of it <u>before</u> such a charge is made. This information might be included in the practice Welcome brochure (see Chapter 1), or it may be printed on the bottom of the statement form.

▶ Divided Payment Plans

In a divided payment plan, the total fee for the planned treatment is to be paid in two or three installments. In most instances a down payment is required before work begins, a payment is made at a certain stage of treatment and the balance is due when the work is completed.

The following is an example of a divided payment plan for a patient who is having a denture made.

- One-third of the fee is paid when preliminary impression is taken. (This is the first step in making the denture.)

- One-third is due when the wax-up is tried in. (This step is about half-way through making the denture.)
- One-third, when the denture is delivered. (This is the last step in the construction of the denture.)

With a divided payment plan, it is essential that the patient make each payment on time. Since payments are tied directly to treatment visits, the dentist may request that you ask for the payment at the *beginning* of the visit.

If the patient fails to make any of these payments on time, be sure the dentist is informed immediately — the dentist may decide to delay the scheduled treatment.

▶ Office Budget Plans

Office budget plans are extended payments, arranged as a convenience to the patient by means of an office contract. When setting up such a plan for the patient, the following information must be taken into consideration.

- Total fee for services.
- Balance to be paid after deduction of the down payment.
- Amount to be financed.
- Number of payments to be made.
- Amount of each payment.
- Date on which each payment is due.

Once this information has been recorded, the budget plan agreement is completed and the patient signs it. The original of this agreement is kept on file in the office and the copy is given to the patient.

When the terms are set for the office budget plan, the patient is given a payment card or booklet showing the balance minus any down payment, the agreed-upon amount of each payment and the due dates (Fig. 8-3). In discussions with the patient, stress that payments are due in the dental office promptly on the scheduled dates.

A file system is used to keep track of when budget plan payments are due. One way to do this is to file the patient budget plan cards chronologically according to the date when the payments are due. An alternative is to file the cards alphabetically and color code them (with file signals) to show when the payments are due.

It is important to follow-up quickly on any budget plan payments that are overdue.

Truth In Lending

When arranging an office budget payment plan, under the following circumstances, it is advisable to complete a *Federal Truth in Lending form* such as the one shown in Figure 8-4.

✓ If there is a **finance charge,** regardless of the number of payments.

✓ If there are **more than four payments** with or without a finance charge.

When this form is used, it should be made out in duplicate with a copy retained with the patient's records.

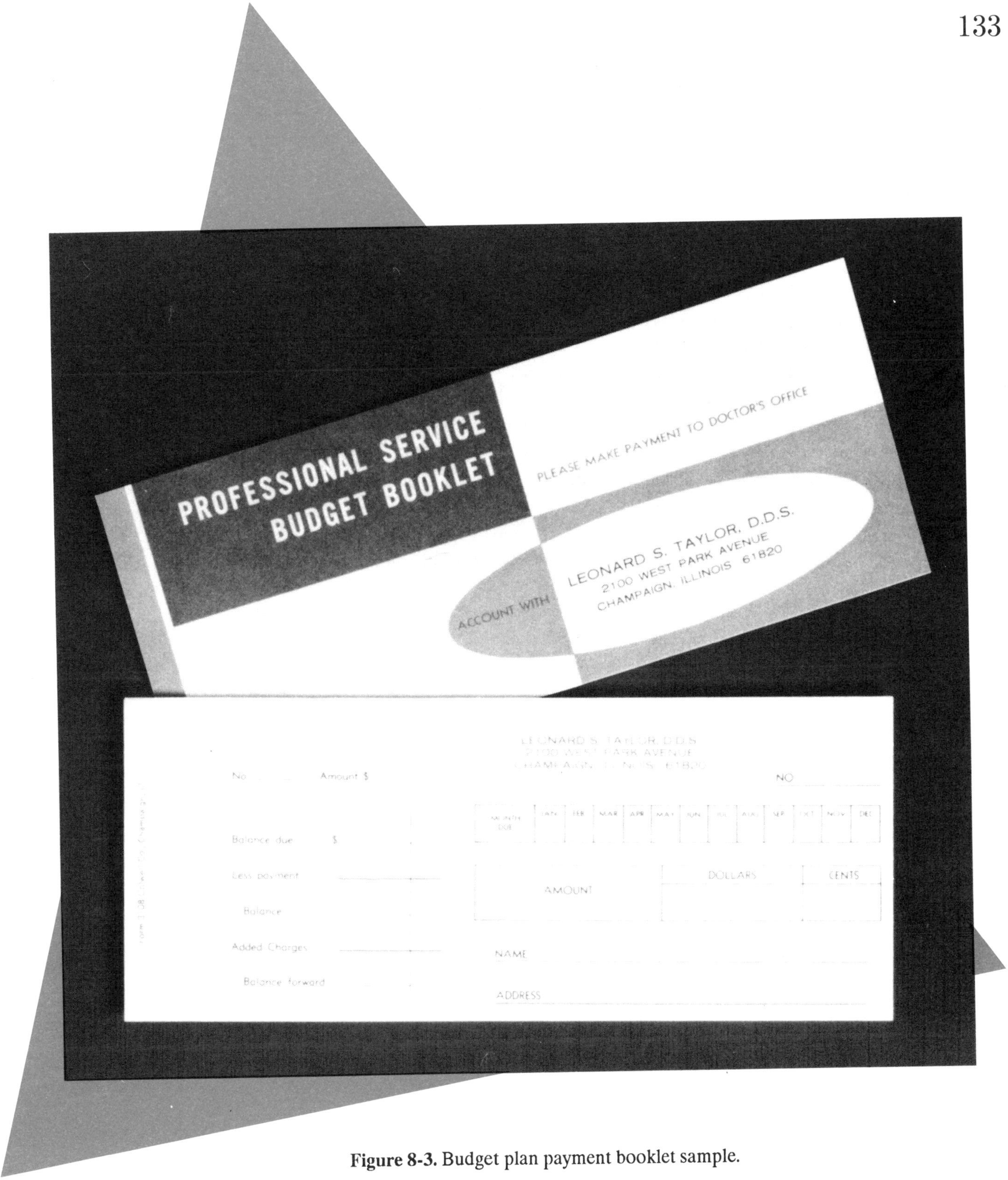

Figure 8-3. Budget plan payment booklet sample.

134

LEONARD S. TAYLOR, D.D.S.
2100 WEST PARK AVENUE
CHAMPAIGN, ILLINOIS 61820

TELEPHONE 351-5400

FEDERAL TRUTH IN LENDING STATEMENT
For professional services rendered

Patient ___ Ruth Gridley (Mrs. James A.) ___

Address ___ 670 Northridge Terrace ___

___ Champaign, IL 61820 ___

Parent _____

1. Fee for Services	$ 1,000.00
2. Total Down Payment	$ 500.00
3. Unpaid Balance	$ 500.00
4. Amount Financed	$ 500.00
5. FINANCE CHARGE	$ –0–
6. Finance Charge Expressed As Annual Percentage Rate	–0–
7. Total Payment Due (4 plus 5)	$ 500.00
8. Total Charges (1 plus 5)	$ 500.00

"Total payment due" (7 above) is payable to ___ Leonard S. Taylor ___
at above office address in ___ 5 ___ monthly installments of $ 100.00.
The first installment is payable on ___ March 1 ___ 19 XX, and
each subsequent payment is due on the same day of each consecutive month
until paid in full.

___ 1/10/xx ___   ___ Ruth Gridley ___
Date   Signature of Patient; Parent if Patient is a Minor

FORM 9402 COLWELL CO., CHAMPAIGN, ILLINOIS

Figure 8-4. Truth in lending form sample.

Computerized Budget Plans

Some accounts receivable programs can also keep track of budget plans. This may include:

- Calculating the amount of each payment.
- Printing the payment booklet.
- Maintaining all necessary account records.
- Generating reports as to when payments are due and which payments are overdue.

MAKING FINANCIAL ARRANGEMENTS

Some form of financial arrangement must be made for every patient. The best time to do this is **before** treatment is provided — and **before** the patient owes money.

Even if the patient has dental insurance, it is still necessary to make financial arrangements with the patient. This includes verifying the amount of coverage and making definite arrangements for the patient's share of the costs.

Making financial arrangements is the process of bringing together the payment plans offered by the dentist and the patient's ability (or willingness) to pay.

This process begins with gathering financial and credit data at the first appointment. It continues through the preparation and presentation of the proposed treatment plan and the cost estimate.

▶ Gathering Financial Data

Financial facts concerning **the person responsible for the account** are gathered on a patient registration form such as the one shown in Figure 1-3 in Chapter 1.

When making arrangements for children of divorced parents, it is particularly important to clearly determine which parent is responsible for payment of the account.

If a mother brings the child for treatment, and says that the father is responsible for the account, verify this with the father and then make the financial arrangements with the father.

Sometimes additional credit references may be needed and the dentist may wish to secure a report from the local credit bureau. When obtained, such information must always be kept in strictest confidence.

If the patient is denied credit because of a negative report, the federal **Fair Credit Reporting Act** requires that the dentist advise the patient of this fact and, on request, must supply the name and address of the agency making the negative report.

▶ Preparing The Treatment Plan And Estimate

After the dentist has examined the patient, a treatment plan may be prepared. This outlines the dentist's treatment recommendations for the patient. When the treatment plan has been completed, an **estimate sheet** should also be prepared for the patient (Fig. 8-5).

This form, which clearly outlines the professional treatment to be rendered and the fees involved, serves as the basis for discussion during the case presentation. It also helps to prevent later misunderstandings about the cost of treatment. The estimate is typed in duplicate so that one copy can be given to the patient and the other copy retained for the office files.

▶ Reaching An Agreement

Financial arrangements must be made with the person who is responsible for payment of the account. These discussions should be held in private and in an unhurried atmosphere. When making these arrangements take into consideration:

- The payment plans offered by the dentist.
- The patient's preferences and ability to pay. (It is better to have the patient make small regular payments as agreed than to miss or be late with larger payments.)
- The period of time over which the treatment and payments will extend.

After an agreement has been reached, a description of the arrangements is noted on the back of the patient's ledger card. Also, if applicable, the necessary forms should be prepared and signed.

COLLECTIONS

▶ The Accounts Receivable Report

The accounts receivable report shows the age of each account. It is a valuable management tool that enables you to identify those accounts that are overdue and require follow-up. These reports include the following categories:

- **Current** — These amounts are for services which have been provided this month. These accounts have not yet received a month-end statement.
- **0-30** — These are accounts which have received one month-end statement and are not yet considered overdue.
- **31-60** — These are accounts which have received two month-end statements and are beginning to be of concern.
- **61-90** — These are accounts which have receive three month-end statements and are definitely overdue.
- **Over 90** — These accounts have received three or more month-end statements and are very overdue!

LEONARD S. TAYLOR, D.D.S.
2100 WEST PARK AVENUE
CHAMPAIGN, ILLINOIS 61820

Telephone 367-6671

| PATIENT'S NAME | Ruth Gridley (Mrs. James A.) | Age | 46 | Date | 1/2/xx |

| ADDRESS | 670 Northridge Terrace | Insurance Co. | Equitable |

Champaign, IL 61820   Policy No. CH-2300

UCR Schedule:

Deductible: $100 family

Annual Maximum: none

Coinsurance %:

Basic Services: 70%

Major Services: 50%

Other:

Exclusions: cosmetic dentistry

Tooth No. or Letter	Description of Services	Dental Code	Doctor's Estimated Fee		Carrier's Resp. *	Patient's Responsibility
	periodontal scaling	04345	$125	00		
14	gold crown	02790	400	00		
19	MOD amalgam restoration	02160	55	00		
20	DO amalgam restoration	02150	45	00		
29	crown (abutment)	06790	400	00		
30	pontic (to replace missing tooth)	06210	400	00		
31	crown (abutment)	06790	400	00		
		TOTALS				

Figure 8-5. Estimate form sample.

Computer Generated Accounts Receivable Report

A computerized bookkeeping system can generate an accounts receivable report, such as the one shown in Figure 8-6, on demand.

These reports may be further specialized to show only delinquent accounts of a specific age and/or amount owed.

Calculating The Account Age For A Manual System

With a pegboard bookkeeping system, this report can be created as necessary. In order to do this, it is necessary to calculate the age of each account.

In calculating the age of the account, follow this basic rule: Any payment made is applied against the earliest outstanding balance until that amount is paid in full. For example:

▸ Any payment made is applied against the earliest outstanding balance until that amount is paid in full.

✓ The Nolan account shows a total balance of $200.
✓ Mrs. Nolan was seen in July and the fee was $100.
✓ Susie Nolan was seen in August and the fee was $25.
✓ Susie Nolan was seen again in September and the fee was $75.
✓ Today, September 15th, Mrs. Nolan made a payment of $125.

To calculate the age of this account, the payment is applied first against the earliest outstanding balance. This would be the $100 from July and then the $25 from August.

This leaves an account balance of $75. This amount is <u>current</u> because these charges were incurred during the present billing period and the Nolans have not yet received a statement for these charges.

▸ **Preventive Account Control**

Most patients are likely to pay their bills; however, many need to be reminded at least once and others require additional follow-up. However, overdue accounts do not age gracefully, and prompt action is required on all outstanding balances. A well-organized account follow-up program is an important tool in these efforts!

▸ Overdue accounts do <u>not</u> age gracefully.

All attempts at collection must be handled tactfully and in keeping with the dentist's wishes, for the dentist does not want to lose patient good-will, or face the threat of legal action because of a careless or angry remark made by an employee.

When planning collections actions, do not always start with the oldest accounts or at the beginning of the alphabet. Instead, review the accounts receivable report to determine which have the largest balances — and which are most likely to respond.

ACCOUNTS RECEIVABLE REPORT
Leonard S. Taylor, D.D.S.

COUNT	NAME	BALANCE	CURRENT	0-30	31-60	61-90	OVER 90
1	Harper	88.00	0.00	88.00	0.00	0.00	0.00
3	Fairchild	177.63	0.00	2.63	175.00	0.00	0.00
6	South	49.00	0.00	49.00	0.00	0.00	0.00
8	Rogers	57.86	0.00	0.86	57.00	0.00	0.00
10	Thompson	306.99	275.00	0.47	0.47	31.05	0.00
12	Martin-Jones	128.78	36.00	1.90	1.88	89.00	0.00
16	Edwards	98.00	0.00	98.00	0.00	0.00	0.00
18	Baker	267.00	149.00	118.00	0.00	0.00	0.00
19	Kilborne	85.26	0.00	1.26	84.00	0.00	0.00
20	Yates	68.00	39.00	29.00	0.00	0.00	0.00
24	Loomis	23.00	0.00	23.00	0.00	0.00	0.00
25	Daniels	257.56	0.00	3.81	3.75	250.00	0.00
27	Miller	117.74	0.00	1.74	116.00	0.00	0.00
29	Greenfield	61.00	0.00	61.00	0.00	0.00	0.00
31	Green	213.00	125.00	88.00	0.00	0.00	0.00
36	Abramson	58.51	7.00	0.76	0.75	50.00	0.00
38	Reed	15.00	0.00	15.00	0.00	0.00	0.00
40	Williams	111.65	0.00	1.65	110.00	0.00	0.00
41	Garrison	128.00	0.00	128.00	0.00	0.00	0.00
42	Parker	77.00	0.00	77.00	0.00	0.00	0.00
45	Yates	197.93	0.00	2.93	195.00	0.00	0.00
47	Blackstone	18.00	0.00	18.00	0.00	0.00	0.00
48	Domber	396.00	125.00	271.00	0.00	0.00	0.00
50	Norman	64.00	64.00	0.00	0.00	0.00	0.00
52	English	82.00	0.00	82.00	0.00	0.00	0.00
55	Nolan	374.00	287.00	87.00	0.00	0.00	0.00
57	Volk	163.04	93.00	1.04	69.00	0.00	0.00
60	Lightner	118.76	0.00	1.76	117.00	0.00	0.00
62	Lawrence	54.00	0.00	54.00	0.00	0.00	0.00
64	Jensen	65.00	0.00	65.00	0.00	0.00	0.00
65	Rockwell	126.00	12.00	114.00	0.00	0.00	0.00
66	Pierce	287.33	287.33	0.00	0.00	0.00	0.00
68	French	40.00	0.00	40.00	0.00	0.00	0.00
70	Agnew	24.45	0.00	0.73	0.72	23.00	0.00
74	Masterson	41.00	0.00	41.00	0.00	0.00	0.00
75	Hardy	115.00	0.00	115.00	0.00	0.00	0.00
77	Clarkson	58.87	0.00	0.87	58.00	0.00	0.00
78	Klein	185.75	0.00	2.75	183.00	0.00	0.00
38 ACCOUNTS		4800.11	1499.33	1686.16	1171.57	443.05	0.00

Figure 8-6. Computer generated accounts receivable report sample.

Collection Follow-Through

The schedule for following through on collections will vary according to the dentist's preferences. The Table "*A Sample Timetable For Collection Follow-up*" shows a typical collection follow-through schedule.

In keeping with these policies you should take prompt action on collections. However, never take unusual or drastic action without specific approval and instructions.

 ## Collection Efforts

The statistics on the Table "*The Relative Effectiveness Of Collection Telephone Calls And Letters*" were supplied by the U.S. Department of Commerce. By comparing the effectiveness of telephone calls versus collection letters, you can see that at 60 days a telephone call is more than twice as effective as a collection letter.

However, notice that at 90 days a telephone call is more than four times as effective as a collection letter — also notice that <u>all</u> collection efforts become less effective with the passage of time!

Making Collection Calls

Making a collection call without doing your homework first is a waste of time and effort! Worse yet, it might cause you to lose money that otherwise would have been collected and to lose the patient as well. The following are the preparatory steps to be taken.

Plan Your Call

It is important that you are clear as to your goals in making this call. For example, you want to:

- **Collect the money due.** (This one is easy to identify, because it is first on almost everyone's list.)
- **Identify the reason for non-payment.** (This is important because, if the patient is dissatisfied, harsh collection steps may prompt legal action. You also need to know the reason for this dissatisfaction so you can take steps to prevent legal action!)
- **Negotiate a payment plan.** (Something is better than nothing, and working out a reasonable payment plan is superior to getting empty promises.)
- **Retain the patient's goodwill.** (Even if you hope the patient will not return again, you really don't want the patient to be angry.)

Review Previous Collection Efforts

All collection efforts should be well documented, and before you make another call you should go over these records. Naturally your plan for this call will be influenced by the success or failure of these previous attempts.

A SAMPLE TIMETABLE FOR COLLECTION FOLLOW-UP	
# DAYS	**COLLECTION ACTION**
0 to 30	Send a statement, this account is not yet overdue.
31 to 60	Mail a second statement with a gently phrased reminder added by hand or typed.
75	Telephone the debtor to determine if there is a problem and how you can help.
90	Send another collection letter or make a follow-up phone call.
105	If you have not received any cooperation or payment, turn the account over for collection. But, before you do this, be sure to get the doctor's permission.

THE RELATIVE EFFECTIVENESS OF COLLECTION TELEPHONE CALLS AND LETTERS		
TIME	LETTER	TELEPHONE
60 days	19%	40%
90 days	6%	25%

Also make certain that you know **who** to contact! You can get in trouble if you talk to the wrong person about an overdue account. (The wrong person is anyone other than the person who is responsible for the account.)

Prepare Your Questions

The manner in which you ask a question often determines the answer you get. As you plan, think backwards. Ask yourself, *"What is the answer I want?"* and then formulate your questions to assure that answer.

Closed-ended questions such as *"Did you send your payment yet?"* and *"Can you have the money here by Friday?"* make the listener feel defensive and will get only yes/no answers.

Instead, use open-ended questions such as *"When may we expect your check?"* or *"How can we help you with this problem?"* You'll be far more successful with this type of question because it gains a more complete response and usually encourages the debtor to be more cooperative.

Have Alternatives Lined Up

Be prepared to offer the debtor alternatives such as using a credit card or setting up an extended payment plan.

Review The Guidelines

The Federal Communications Commission has established guidelines for making collection calls. These are outlined in the Table *"Guidelines Regarding Collection Calls."*

Review these guidelines before you call — and then follow them carefully!

GUIDELINES REGARDING COLLECTION CALLS

CALLS AT ODD HOURS OF THE DAY OR NIGHT

- The law prohibits collection calls made at hours known to be other than the **normal waking hours** of the called party. In most situations, this is between 8 am and 9 pm.

REPEATED CALLS

- Generally, scheduling more than one call per week to the debtor to discuss the amount owed is considered inappropriate. (More than one call per week is considered harassment.)
- Call backs, left word to call, follow-ups of promises are **excluded.** So, too, are instances where the debtor requests an additional call, such as a request to call back in the evening, at home.

CALLS TO PLACES OF EMPLOYMENT

- A request by an **employer** that no further calls be made to the employee (debtor) at the place of business *must* be honored.
- Requests by the debtor that no further calls be made to his place of employment should also be honored.

CALLS TO THIRD PARTIES

- Calls to "third parties" should generally be made only for the purpose of locating the debtor or when the debtor cannot be contacted directly by telephone. Requests by third parties that no further calls be received must be honored.
- Never indicate to the third party that you are calling about an overdue bill; however, you may say that it is a *"financial matter."*

CALLS ASSERTING LEGAL ACTION

- It is not permissible to make such statements just to frighten the debtor into paying. However, it is acceptable to advise the debtor of the possible consequences of continued failure to satisfy the debt.
- For example, if you assert that the debtor's credit rating will be hurt, but don't report the account to the credit bureau, this threat is made to frighten the debtor — and is not permissible.
- On the other hand, if you intend taking the debtor into small claims court, it is important to inform him of this possibility.

Make The Call

The steps outlined in the Table "*Five Steps To Making Successful Collection Calls*" will help you make these collection calls. Very few people really like to make these calls; however with proper preparation you can do it effectively!

FIVE STEPS TO MAKING SUCCESSFUL COLLECTION CALLS	
STEP 1:	**IDENTIFY YOURSELF AND YOUR PRACTICE** Say this clearly, so there is no question as to who is calling, and speak in a confident tone of voice. Remember, you are a professional and you have a job to do. For example, "*Good morning Mr. Smith, this is Sue Jackson. I'm calling from Dr. Taylor's office.*"
STEP 2:	**GIVE YOUR REASON FOR CALLING** Your tone of voice is very important as you state the reason for your call. You don't want to sound angry or anxious. You do want to sound direct and businesslike. For example, "*I'm calling about your overdue account.*"
STEP 3:	**MAKE A STRATEGIC PAUSE** Six seconds of silence at this point is the first step to putting the responsibility of the collections call on the debtor. For example, *SAY NOTHING. WAIT FOR MR. SMITH TO RESPOND!*
STEP 4:	**WORK OUT A SOLUTION** Depending upon Mr. Smith's response, ask the appropriate questions based on your planning. Remember that these questions are going to help you achieve your goals for this call. (Also, remember to stay cool, no matter how irate Mr. Smith may be.) For example, "*Mr. Smith, we'd be happy to help you by setting up a payment plan. How much could you pay each week?*"
STEP 5:	**CONCLUDE THE CALL** In finishing the call, always let the debtor know that some action is about to be taken on your part. Usually this is recording the agreement; however, it could be turning the account over for collection if you were unable to reach any agreement. For example, "*Mr. Smith, I'm glad we could work out a payment plan to help you. We'll expect your first check for $25 this Friday and then another check each Friday over the next two months. Thank you.*"

▶ Collection Letters

There are times when a collection letter is necessary. In these situations, a personal letter is more effective than a form letter (Figs. 8-7 and 8-8).

In writing a collection letter there is no point in trying to hide the message in flowery double-talk. The message should be clear and to the point — without being offensive. The patient who receives a collection letter knows that the account is overdue and is well aware of why the letter is being sent.

All collection letters should be phrased in firm, positive, businesslike terms. They should make every effort to persuade the patient to want to pay the debt, to encourage even a partial payment, and to enable the patient to save face while doing so.

Collection letters may be signed by the dentist, or by the secretarial assistant. When the secretarial assistant signs the letter, the information under the signature should give his or her name and title as well as the dentist's name. For example, *"Mary Wells, C.D.A., Secretarial Assistant to Leonard Taylor, D.D.S."*

▶ Skip Tracing

If a statement is returned marked *"Moved — No Forwarding Address,"* the account can be considered a **skip.** This calls for immediate action to trace the individual. There are several possible steps in tracing skips.

- Call the telephone number you have listed on the record. The patient may have transferred the old number, or you may be given a new number.
- If you have the name of a relative, friend or other reference, they may be able to give you information.
- Check the patient's place of employment. While they may not give you his address, it is possible they will relay a message.
- Place the words *"address correction requested"* below the return address on the envelope. This indicates you want to know where the mail is being delivered other than the address listed. For a fee, the post office will make a search, forward the mail to the new address, and inform you of this new address.
- Send a registered letter, with a return receipt requested. This should be sent in a plain envelope with no return address so that the patient will not see the return address and refuse to accept the letter.

▶ Collection Agencies

▶ Never turn an account over for collection without the doctor's permission.

The final decision about turning cases over to a collection agency must be the dentist's. However, when unpaid accounts are to be referred to a collector, this should be done while there is still hope of settlement.

LEONARD S. TAYLOR, D.D.S.

June 1, 19XX

Mr. Wayne Hardison
578 Dogwood Drive
Urbana, IL 61821

Dear Mr. Hardison:

Our records show that your account of $168 is now more than 90 days overdue — and that you have failed to respond to our efforts to work out an acceptable payment plan.

Because I know it will damage your credit rating in the community, I am reluctant to turn this account over to a collection agency. However unless payment in full is received by June 10th, I will be forced to turn your account over to the ABC Collection Agency for immediate action.

I hope we can resolve this problem without having to take this step.

Sincerely,

Leonard S. Taylor, D.D.S.

Leonard S. Taylor, D.D.S.

LST/mw

2100 WEST PARK AVENUE   CHAMPAIGN, ILLINOIS 61820   TELEPHONE 351-5400

Figure 8-7. Collection letter #1 sample.

146

LEONARD S. TAYLOR, D.D.S.

May 1, 19XX

Mr. Wayne Hardison
578 Dogwood Drive
Urbana, IL 61821

Dear Mr. Hardison:

Is something wrong? Our records show that your account of $168 is now more than 60 days overdue.

We want to make certain that there hasn't been a mistake. Please help by checking the appropriate information below and returning this to us in the enclosed envelope.

If you are having a problem paying this account, please telephone me and I will be happy to work out a new payment plan for you.

Thank you.

Sincerely,

Mary Wells, C. D. A.

Mary Wells, C.D.A.,
Secretarial Assistant to
Leonard S. Taylor, D.D.S.

- -

_____ I paid this amount on _____ with check # _____.

_____ My check is enclosed for $168.

_____ My check is enclosed for $_____.
I will send the balance by _____.

_____   _____
  (date)   (signature)

2100 WEST PARK AVENUE   CHAMPAIGN, ILLINOIS 61820   TELEPHONE 351-5400

Figure 8-8. Collection letter #2 sample.

Make every effort to collect an account without having to resort to turning it over to an agency. Turning the account over to the agency will cost the practice 30% to 50% of the amount collected. It will also alienate, and irritate, the patient. This could cause a patient to think about suing the doctor to "get even."

- Notify patients in writing that if they don't make payment, or make an arrangement, the account will be turned over to a collection agency.
- Give the patient a reasonable amount of time to respond — usually 10 days to two weeks.
- Give the agency all the information you have which may be helpful and keep them posted on any new developments. Cooperate with the collector and call promptly if the patient makes payment directly to the practice.

A collection agency will receive from the patient only the amount of the fee for dental care. No fee for their services will be added. The agency is paid by keeping a percentage of the amount collected from the patient.

Usually on a monthly basis, the agency will report the results of its efforts and send a check for the net amount due the dentist.

▶ Small Claims Court

Small claims court is another option for collecting small overdue accounts. It is not always necessary for the doctor to appear in court. Instead, it is possible to arrange to have someone else, such as an employee, to handle the claim. The following are guidelines to be followed when taking a case into small claims court.

Small Claims Only

The amount of your claim must be under the limit established in your locale. Maximum claims range from $300 to $5,000. However, the majority of states allow only a maximum of $1,000.

The Defendant

In these cases the person you are trying to collect from is the **defendant**. The person who is trying to collect is the **plaintiff**.

Before you can file your case in small claims court, you must have the full legal name and current mailing address of the defendant. This is necessary so that the court can notify the defendant of the legal action. Remember, if you can't find the defendant, chances are that the court can't either.

Filing The Claim

In most states you must file the claim in the **jurisdiction** (city or county) where the defendant lives. This means that if the defendant lives in another part of the state, you must travel there.

To file the claim, go to the small claims court, complete the necessary paperwork and pay your filing fee. These fees vary from less than $4 to more than $20.

Once you've done this, a date is set for the "hearing" or "trial" and the papers will be served to the defendant. However, the defendant may request a postponement.

Be Prepared

It is important to document your case carefully. This means that you must be prepared to show how much the defendant owes and the efforts that have been made to collect this amount.

For example, if you have a signed financial agreement this could be introduced as evidence. Information presented must not reveal any clinical information concerning the patient's condition or treatment.

The Judgment

The judge will hear the case and issue a ruling — even if the defendant fails to attend the hearing. If you win, a **judgment** will be issued stating that the defendant owes you a certain amount of money.

This generally includes the original amount owed plus court costs, such as your filing fee. It does not include anything for the value of your time in bringing the case to court.

Collecting The Judgment

Even if you win the case, the court will not act as your collection agent. This means that you still must collect the amount owed.

If the defendant does not pay within a reasonable time, inform the court clerk and you'll be instructed as to what steps to take next. For example, a lien may be placed against the defendant's property; however, you can't collect anything until the defendant decides to sell that property.

Chapter

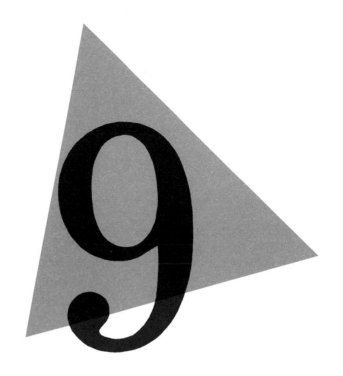

INVENTORY CONTROL AND PURCHASING

LEARNING GOALS

The student will be able to:

▶ Define: rate of use, order point, shelf life, purchase order, packing slip, invoice and back order.

▶ List the supplies needed for a card-file inventory system and describe the use of each.

▶ Demonstrate determining the reorder point for a supply item.

▶ Demonstrate establishing the order quantity for a supply item.

▶ List three guidelines for ordering supplies.

▶ Describe the process of stocking new supplies.

OVERVIEW OF INVENTORY CONTROL AND PURCHASING

Running out of any supply can create an unnecessary crisis, such as being unable to complete a patient's treatment because the needed supplies were not readily available!

However, effective inventory control can eliminate this problem (Fig. 9-1). Also, a well-managed purchasing system can help reduce waste and control practice costs.

The dentist will establish policies for the management of purchasing and inventory control. Then, a member of the business office staff is assigned the responsibility of carrying out these policies while ordering supplies and maintaining the inventory system.

Although one person has the primary responsibility for this, all other staff members are expected to cooperate by promptly reporting when supplies reach the reorder point.

▶ Running out of any supply can create an unnecessary crisis!

▶ Computerized Inventory Control

Computerized systems are available for inventory control; however, these are used primarily for high volume applications such as retail stores and warehouses.

At this time, a well organized manual system is still the most cost effective inventory control method for the dental office.

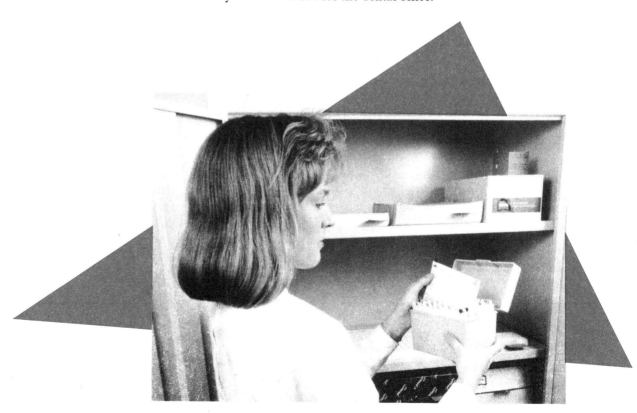

Figure 9-1. Effective inventory control can prevent an unnecessary crisis and save the practice money.

ESTABLISHING AN
INVENTORY CONTROL SYSTEM

When establishing an inventory system, it is necessary to determine the reorder point and the order quantity for each item stocked (Fig 9-2).

✓ The **reorder point** is the minimum quantity of a given item which is an adequate reserve for that product. This point is marked in the current inventory. When it is reached, it is time to reorder the product.

✓ The **order quantity** is the optimal amount of a given item to be purchased at one time. Several factors are taken into consideration so that supplies are purchased at the best possible price.

▶ The order quantity is the optimal amount of a given item to be purchased at one time.

NAME OF PRODUCT ___Patient Towels___

1. APPROXIMATE RATE OF USE

    20 per day; 100 per week

2. SHELF LIFE OF PRODUCT

    unlimited

3. AMOUNT OF STORAGE SPACE REQUIRED

    bulky to store; must be dry

4. TIME LAPSE BETWEEN ORDERING & RECEIVING PRODUCT

    allow two weeks

5. OTHER FACTORS

    Use rate varies -- allow for increase
    Watch for specials

6. BEST QUANTITY PURCHASE RATE   (500 per carton)

    1 carton $23.00
    4 cartons $75.00

REORDER POINT $\frac{1}{2}$ carton   ORDER QUANTITY 4 cartons

---

Figure 9-2. The steps in establishing reorder point and order quantity.

> ### Determining The Reorder Point

The reorder point is based on these three factors:

- The **rate of use:** How much of the product is used within a given period of time.
- The **lead time:** The time lapse between ordering and receiving the product.
- A **margin of safety:** The time allowed to accommodate any delay in delivery or a sudden increase in use.

To see how this works, lets look at the steps in determining the rate of use and reorder point for welcome brochures in Dr. Taylor's practice.

The Rate Of Use

A welcome brochure is given to each new patient, and Dr. Taylor sees about 10 new patients per week.

To determine the rate of use, it is only necessary to count the number of new patient visits listed in the appointment book for two or three weeks and divide to establish the average number per week.

In addition, about 10 brochures per week are given to patients for their friends (who might be prospective new patients) and to other practice visitors. This puts the current rate of use at approximately 20 brochures per week and 80 per month.

Lead Time

These brochures are custom printed and it usually takes two weeks, or less, to get a new supply. Therefore, the lead time is two weeks. Based on the current rate of use, 40 brochures would be a two week supply.

A Margin Of Safety

> A margin of safety protects against a sudden increase in the rate of use and/or unexpected delays in receiving the new supply.

A margin of safety protects against a sudden increase in the rate of use and/or unexpected delays in receiving the new supply. To be really safe, particularly since Dr. Taylor's practice continues to grow, the reorder point for welcome brochures is set at 50.

> ### Determining The Order Quantity

To determine the order quantity for an item it is necessary to review the following factors. As we look at them, let's determine the order quantity for welcome brochures.

The Rate Of Use

Knowing the rate of use is important. It is inefficient, and usually not cost effective, to reorder a supply too frequently. On the other hand, it is wasteful to have a large stock of an infrequently used item. We have already established that the brochures are used at the rate of 20 per week or 80 per month.

Storage Space Requirements

If storage space is limited, it is not a good idea to order large quantities of a bulky item such as paper towels. Welcome brochures are not bulky, so this is not a concern for this product.

The Shelf Life

Some products, such as x-ray film and certain antibiotics, deteriorate with age and should not be used after the expiration date shown on the package. These products are said to have a limited **Shelf life.** Welcome brochures do not have a limited shelf life, so this is not a concern for this product.

The Probability Of Continued Use

When one product is replaced by an improved one, the doctor probably will not continue to use the older product. For example, the dentist may not want to stock up on one type of impression material when it looks as if a newer one will work better.

Dr. Taylor definitely plans to continue using welcome brochures, and he likes to update these brochures periodically. Therefore, he does not want to buy a supply that will last for years.

Price Breaks For Quantity Purchase

1. The hypothetical price range for these brochures is:

    100 for $25
    200 for $40
    500 for $95

2. Based on the current rate of use:

    100 brochures will last two months
    200 will last four months
    500 will last 10 months

3. Since Dr. Taylor recently updated the welcome brochure, he wants to take advantage of the price break for purchasing 500 at a time.

    Therefore, the order quantity for this product is 500.

THE PARTS OF A CARD-FILE INVENTORY SYSTEM

The key to effective inventory control is to establish a simple, easy-to-use system, and routinely follow it. The most frequently used method is a card-file inventory system which consists of the following parts.

▶ The Inventory Control Card

The basis of this system is the use of 4" x 6" inventory and order control cards (Fig.9-3). One of these cards is filled out for each important supply item. The following basic information is noted on each supply card:

✓ The name of the product
✓ The order quantity
✓ The reorder point
✓ The order source

When noting the order source, make a complete entry so that you don't need to take time to look up the address or telephone number.

Cross-reference cards are needed for materials that are sometimes referred to by brand name and sometimes by generic description. For example, amalgam (which is the generic name for silver restoration material) may also be specified by a brand name.

ORDER	(ITEM NAME) Reply Envelopes									ON ORDER

ORDER QUANTITY _2000_   REORDER POINT _500_

ORDER	QTY	REC'D	COST	PREPAID	ON ACCT	ORDER	QTY	REC'D	COST	PREPAID	ON ACCT

INVENTORY COUNT

	JAN	FEB	MAR	APR	MAY	JUNE	JULY	AUG	SEPT	OCT	NOV	DEC
19 ___												
19 ___												

ORDER SOURCE   **UNIT PRICE**

Colwell Systems Inc.

201 Kenyon Road

Champaign, IL 61820

FORM 2450 COLWELL CO., CHAMPAIGN, ILLINOIS

Figure 9-3. Inventory control card sample.

The File Box And Index

The cards are filed alphabetically and stored in a file box. Alphabetical indexing dividers are used to speed finding and filing cards.

If there are so many cards that a single box would be too crowded, the cards are divided into two sets: one for clinical materials and the second for office supplies. The cards are then stored in separate file boxes with separate indexing dividers.

Metal File Signals

Colored metal file signals are used to indicate when supplies need to be ordered and/or when they are on order.

✓ A metal file signal is placed on the **upper left corner** of the card when a supply needs to be ordered.
✓ The file signal is moved to the **upper right corner** of the card to indicate that the supply has been ordered.
✓ When the supply is received, the file signal is removed.

Red Flag Reorder Tags

These red paper tags are used to mark the reorder point of a supply. The name of the supply and the reorder point are written on the red flag before it is put into use (Fig. 9-4).

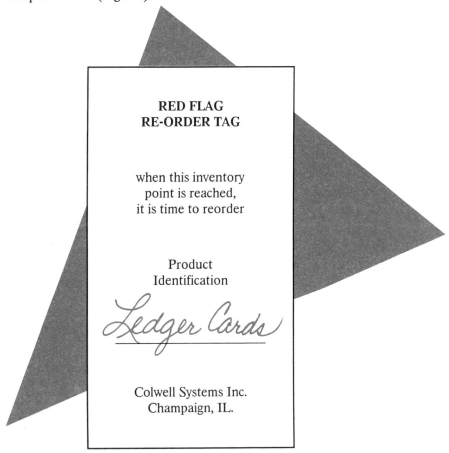

**RED FLAG
RE-ORDER TAG**

when this inventory
point is reached,
it is time to reorder

Product
Identification

Ledger Cards

Colwell Systems Inc.
Champaign, IL.

Figure 9-4. A red flag is used to mark the reorder point.

When the reorder point is reached, the flag is removed and given to the person in charge of ordering supplies. Once the reorder point has been reached, the new supply should be ordered promptly.

The flag is placed in the appropriate spot to mark the reorder point for each item. For example:

- If the reorder point for patient charts is 100, a red flag is placed in the stack of charts about 100 up from the bottom of the stack.
- Boxed supplies, such as x-ray film, may have the tag attached with a rubber band around the minimum quantity.
- For bulky items, the tag may be taped to the appropriate box.

HOW TO USE THE SYSTEM

1. Complete a card for each major supply and file the cards alphabetically in the appropriate file box.

2. Complete a red flag for each item and mark the reorder point on all current supplies.

3. When a supply reaches the reorder point, the red flag is removed and given to the person responsible for ordering supplies.

4. When a supply needs to be ordered, place a colored tab over the "order" section. (This file signal can also be used to hold the red flag with the inventory card until the new supply is received.)

5. Place orders promptly.

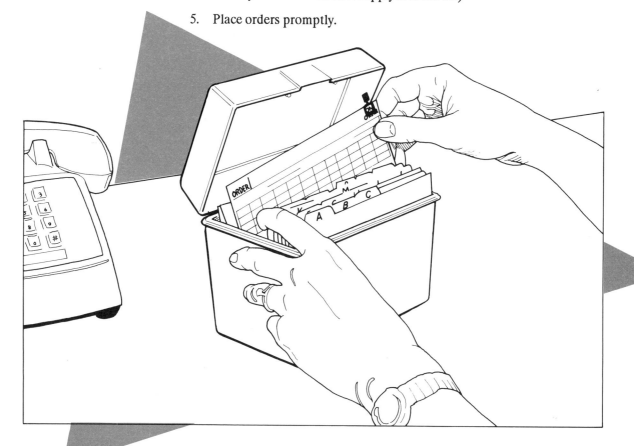

Figure 9-5. A file signal on the right corner indicates that the supply has been ordered.

6. When the order is placed, note the date and quantity ordered and move the colored tab to the "on order" position (Fig. 9-5).

7. When the supply is received, note the date and quantity. Also, remove the file signal and the red flag.

8. Stock the supplies carefully and use the red flag to once again mark the reorder point.

GUIDELINES FOR ORDERING SUPPLIES

▶ Be Prepared

Review the inventory and ask if the dentist has any requests before the sales representative is due to call, or before you are ready to phone or mail an order.

▶ Be Specific

Know what you need and how much you need of it . When placing an order, it is helpful to have the catalog in front of you. Be prepared to provide or verify the following information:

- The catalog number (if ordering by phone, it also helps to note the catalog page number).
- Descriptive details (including brand names or style information).
- The quantity to be ordered.
- Pricing information.

▶ Purchase Orders

A large group practice may issue purchase orders to authorize the purchase of supplies. In this situation, have the purchase order and number ready before calling the supplier.

A **purchase order** is a form authorizing the purchase of specific supplies from a specific supplier. These forms are numbered and, when placing an order, the supplier may refer to the purchase order number.

▶ Handling Back Orders

If the supplier cannot make prompt shipment of an item, it will be back ordered. (A **back order** is a notification that an item is out of stock or not currently available.)

The back order notice should include an estimate as to when the product will be available and delivered. If you cannot wait until this future date, it is necessary to purchase the supply elsewhere and notify the original supplier that you want to cancel the order for this item.

▶ Be Alert

Be on the lookout for specials and authentic savings. However, a bargain on something you don't need or use — is no bargain! Before placing an order, review the current price and take advantage of any promotional sales, seasonal savings or convention specials.

▶ Be Informed

Just as the dentist will want to keep abreast of new product information, you should be alert for new products and ideas that can make your business office responsibilities easier to manage. When journals and catalogs come in, review them and look for ideas that can be adapted for your use.

STORING SUPPLIES

▶ Organizing The Storage Area

1. Good supply control requires organized storage, and the storage area should be cool, dry, clean and well-lighted.

2. Keep a fire extinguisher in the storage area. Check the dial on it periodically to be certain that it is properly charged.

3. Do not allow trash and clutter to accumulate. They are a fire hazard.

4. Store bulky or heavy and frequently-used items near the floor where they can be easily reached.

5. Store small, or related items, together in boxes or bins.

6. Store materials according to the manufacturer's directions. For example:

   * Refrigeration for some antibiotics.
   * A locked cabinet for narcotics.
   * Cool, dry storage for envelopes and paper products.

7. Clearly label all shelves and bins. This makes it easier to find things — particularly for new employees.

   It also enables you to quickly spot when an item is completely out of stock.

▶ Stocking Fresh Supplies

1. When an order is received and unpacked, check the contents against the invoice or packing slip to be sure that the correct materials came in and in the proper quantities.

   A **packing slip** is an itemized listing of the goods shipped. It does not contain pricing information.

   An **invoice** is an itemized listing of the goods shipped which includes pricing information. The invoice will be used when paying for the supplies.

2. Then locate the inventory control cards. For each item:

   * Remove the metal file signal.
   * Enter the date, the quantities received and the newest prices.
   * Return the cards to their appropriate place in the file.

3. Place the red flag reorder tag at the reorder point of the new supplies (Fig. 9-6).

4. Place the fresh supplies behind the older ones.

▶ Fresh supplies are always placed behind the older ones.

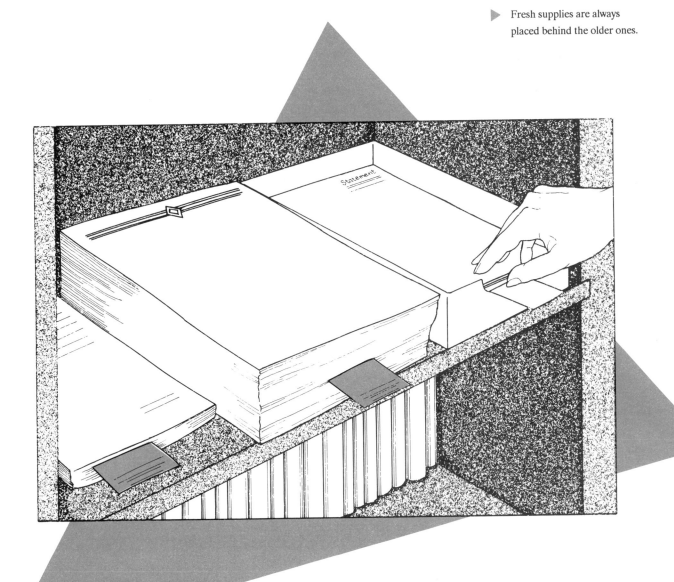

Figure 9-6. When stocking fresh supplies, place the red flag to mark the reorder point.

Chapter

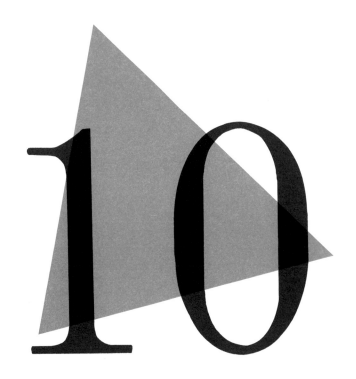

ACCOUNTS PAYABLE BOOKKEEPING

LEARNING GOALS

The student will be able to:

▶ Describe accounts payable bookkeeping.
▶ Describe the steps involved in preparing to pay bills and in maintaining expense documentation.
▶ Define: consummables, predating, postdating, payee, bank statement, reconcile, deposits in transit.
▶ Differentiate between gross pay and net pay.
▶ Identify the payroll taxes which are deducted from an employee's earnings and those which the employer must pay.
▶ Demonstrate writing checks using a pegboard checkwriting system.
▶ Demonstrate reconciling a simulated bank statement.

162

Accounts payable bookkeeping is the management, verification, and prompt payment of the practice expenses for supplies, payroll, rent and similar costs (Fig. 10-1). These expenses represent **overhead**, or the dentist's cost of doing business.

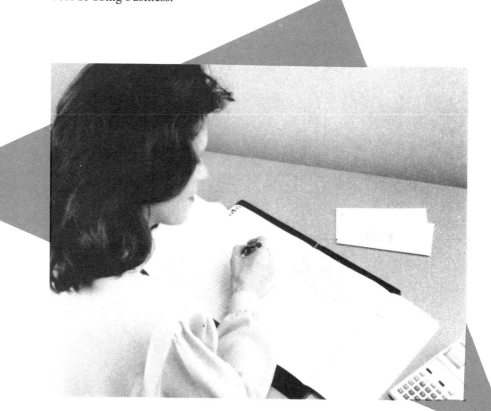

Figure 10-1. Accounts payable bookkeeping is the management, verification and prompt payment of practice expenses.

▶ Practice expenses must be managed in a business-like manner.

▶ To Be Paid

All bills awaiting payment should be stored in an accounts payable folder. Packing slips, invoices, and statements are placed in this **To Be Paid** file as they are received.

▶ Preparing To Pay Bills

Bills offering a discount for prompt payment should be paid at once. Others are usually paid about the 10th and 25th of the month.

- At this time, remove all papers from the accounts payable folder and organize them by vendor.
- If a statement covers several invoices received during the month, check each invoice against its listing on the statement.
- When the invoices and their covering statement have been verified, staple the invoices to the back of the statement.
- The dentist may want to review these bills before you write the checks. Or, you may be asked to organize the bills so that someone else can write and sign the checks.

► **Expense Documentation**

Once a bill or statement has been paid, it is marked with the date and check number. Then it is filed in the folder according to its applicable category. For example, a folder for utilities will hold the gas, electric and water bills.

Expenses are summarized by categories to provide important management data. Samples of commonly used catagories are shown in the Table *"Office Expense Categories."*

OFFICE EXPENSE CATEGORIES	
● **Professional Supplies:** Drugs, supplies and small instruments which are purchased regularly.	● **Laboratory Fees:** Amounts paid to commercial laboratories or costs charged against an "in-office" laboratory.
● **Salaries:** Enter the actual amount of each payroll check (after deductions), plus all checks written to the state and Federal governments in payment of payroll taxes.	● **Rent, Upkeep of Office:** This includes rent, heat, cleaning, minor repairs and redecorating.
● **Electricity, Gas, and Water:** These may also be grouped together as utilities (electricity, gas and water), with telephone being handled as a separate category.	● **Office Supplies:** Enter here stationery, record and bookkeeping supplies, printing, copy-machine supplies, telephone and postage.
● **Insurance, Taxes:** Insurance on equipment, liability, professional malpractice. The taxes included here are personal property taxes on equipment, and professional licenses.	● **Dues, Books, and Journals:** This includes membership in professional organizations, plus the cost of professional journals and reference books.
● **Auto Upkeep:** Enter all operating costs on a car used for professional purposes. (Depreciation is added at the end of the year.) Only that portion of car expenses which is for professional use may be deducted.	● **Travel:** Travel is for consultations, conventions, and professional meetings. This includes items such as transportion, hotels and meals.
● **Laundry, Cleaning:** These are only the laundry and dry cleaning expenses (such as towels and uniforms) which are directly related to the practice.	● **Goodwill:** Goodwill covers expenses, such as sending flowers to a patient, that can be established as benefiting the earning power of the practice.
● **Miscellaneous:** This is a general category for practice expenses which do not fit into the other categories. Whenever possible, expenses should be entered under a more specific category.	● **Sundry:** This category is for expenses that are <u>not</u> costs of doing business but which were paid from the office account.

164

▶ The Depreciation Schedule

Supplies and minor pieces of equipment which are used up fairly quickly are known as **consummables.** These are handled as practice expenses.

Major purchases, such as dental equipment or a computer, must be written-off over a period of time. This process is called **depreciation** and it represents the value that is lost through wear or obsolescence. The practice accountant usually establishes and maintains the depreciation schedule.

▶ The Annual Expense Summary

After the accuracy of the entries have been verified, totals of earnings and costs are carried forward to the annual report.

PAYROLL TAXES AND RECORDS

Federal regulations require that an employer make certain deductions from an employee's pay, and that the employer also pay certain payroll taxes. These requirements are explained in **Circular E, The Employer's Tax Guide,** which is issued annually by the Internal Revenue Service.

State taxes must also be paid, and the appropriate state publication should be consulted for this information. If you are responsible for preparing payroll checks and maintaining payroll records, take time to review these publications and follow their instructions very carefully.

▶ Government Reports

The federal and state governments require the employer to deposit all taxes withheld, plus the employer's contributions, on a regular basis. (Circular E contains a schedule of the forms and their due dates.)

All government reports must be filled out exactly and neatly. These must always be filed **on time** — there is a penalty for late reports.

A copy of all reports should be kept with the office records. These, and back payroll records, should be retained with other valuable office papers for a period of at least four years after the taxes involved have been paid.

▶ Payroll Records

The government requires that the employer keep records regarding the amounts paid to each employee and the amounts deducted (Fig. 10-2). This means that complete and accurate employee summaries should be kept up-to-date.

A separate payroll sheet should be maintained for each employee. The heading of this form shows the employee's name, address, social security number, and the number of exemptions claimed.

For each pay period, the dates and **gross pay** (total amount earned) are entered. Also, the amounts to be withheld for taxes are calculated and the net pay is recorded. (**Net pay** is the amount received after deductions have been subtracted.)

The accuracy of these entries should be verified by adding the total of all deductions to the net pay. The resulting sum should equal the amount of the gross pay.

▶ Government reports must be filed on time.

NAME	Mary Wells, C.D.A.						SOC. SEC. NO.		482-31-4957
ADDRESS	210 West Bradley, Champaign			TEL. 351-0148			NO. OF EXEMPTIONS		1

DATE 19 XX	GROSS PAY		DEDUCTIONS					NET PAY		DATE 19	GROSS PAY		DEDUCTIONS					NET PAY	
			FICA		INC TAX								FICA		INC TAX				
JAN 8	320	00	22	88	40	00		257	12	JULY									
15	320	00	22	88	40	00		257	12										
22	320	00	22	88	40	00		257	12										
29	320	00	22	88	40	00		257	12	← AMOUNT IN PAYCHECK									
TOTAL JANUARY	1280	00	91	52	160	00		1028	48	TOTAL JULY									
FEB										AUG									
										THE EMPLOYEE PAYS THIS TAX									
										THE EMPLOYER MUST MAKE A MATCHING CONTRIBUTION									
TOTAL FEBRUARY	AMOUNT ACTUALLY EARNED									TOTAL AUGUST									
MARCH										SEPT									
TOTAL MARCH										TOTAL SEPT									
TOTAL 1ST QTR										TOTAL 3RD QTR									
APRIL										OCT									
TOTAL APRIL										TOTAL OCTOBER									
MAY										NOV									
TOTAL MAY										TOTAL NOVEMBER									
JUNE										DEC									
TOTAL JUNE										TOTAL DECEMBER									
TOTAL 2ND QTR										TOTAL 4TH QTR									
			TOTALS FOR THE YEAR 19																

FORM 7247 COLWELL CO., CHAMPAIGN, ILLINOIS

Figure 10-2. Payroll record sample.

▶ Payroll Deductions

Income Tax Withholding

All employees must pay federal income tax and file a tax return. A portion of this tax is deducted from each paycheck. Income tax is strictly an employee tax (the employer does not make any matching contribution), and the amount withheld depends upon the number of exemptions claimed by the employee.

Each employee must complete a **Withholding Exemption Certification** (W-4 form) which authorizes the employer to deduct the tax and indicates the number of exemptions which the employee is claiming.

This form must be completed when a new employee starts work. It is not completed before the first wage payment, taxes are withheld as if the employee is single, with no withholding allowance.

Wage and tax statements (W-2 forms) showing total earnings and taxes withheld for the calendar year must be given to employees not later than January 31 of the following year.

Social Security

Under the **Federal Insurance Contributions Act** (FICA), commonly known as Social Security, the employer is required to deduct a certain percentage of the employee's gross pay. This is a fixed amount regardless of the number of exemptions.

The employer is also required to make a matching contribution. For example, for every dollar withheld from the employee's pay for Social Security, the employer also contributes a dollar.

To assure that payments are accurately credited to the employee's social security account, it is essential that the Social Security Administration be notified of any change of name. This notification is the employee's responsibility and should be handled immediately after marriage or other change of name.

Federal And State Unemployment Tax

The employer is required to make contributions to state and federal funds to cover the cost of unemployment benefits paid out within that state.

This is usually referred to as *FUTA*, and it is strictly an employer tax. This tax <u>may not</u> be deducted from the employee's pay.

Workers' Compensation

Under state law, the employer is also required to contribute to workers' compensation to cover the medical expenses for employees who are injured on the job. This, too, is an employer tax and <u>may not</u> be deducted from the employee's pay.

The accuracy of these figures is extremely important because they form the basis of practice tax returns and other financial reports. Also, they could be subject to examination in years to come. Therefore, it is particularly important that all entries here be neat and complete.

THE PETTY CASH FUND

Large bills should always be paid by check; however, a petty cash fund may be used to pay minor bills, such as postage due or laundry delivered. Petty cash is <u>not</u> the same as the change fund which is explained in Chapter 6.

The amount of the petty cash fund is limited (usually not more than $50) and the funds are kept in small bills and coins so that it is possible to make exact change. Each withdrawal must be indicated by voucher or note explaining the purpose of the expenditure (Fig. 10-3). If possible, a receipt should be attached to the voucher.

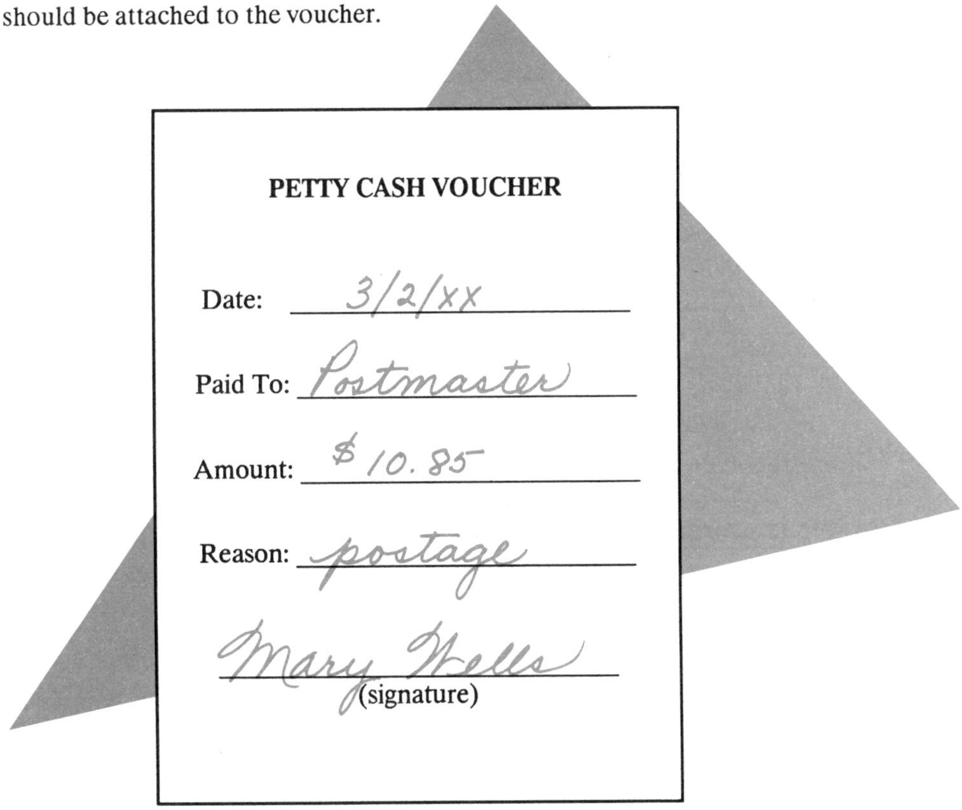

PETTY CASH VOUCHER

Date: *3/2/xx*

Paid To: *Postmaster*

Amount: *$10.85*

Reason: *postage*

Mary Wells
(signature)

Figure 10-3. Petty cash voucher sample.

► Replenishing Petty Cash

The petty cash fund should be balanced and replenished about once a month. To do this follow these steps:

- Total all vouchers and add this figure to the cash on hand. If the fund is in balance, with all withdrawals accounted for, this should equal the original amount of the fund.
- Staple all vouchers and attached receipts together, then note the total amount and the date. Petty cash expenses are usually listed along with office supplies and the vouchers are placed in the appropriate file folder.
- Write a check for the amount needed to bring the fund back to the original amount. The check is cashed (be sure to get small bills) and the money placed back in the petty cash fund.

167

CHECK WRITING

Checks must be written properly in order to make fraudulent alteration or endorsement difficult. The following are the basic rules of check writing.

▶ The Entries Must Be Accurate And Complete

Always be certain that the check stub or check register information is filled out completely and accurately. Unless you are using a pegboard, one-write system, or a computer, the check stub should be completed *before* you write the check.

▶ Use Ink

Checks are written in ink, by typewriter, or printed by the computer. They are never written in pencil.

A **check-writer** is a machine which is used to emboss the amount of the check into the fiber of the paper. The purpose of this is to prevent alterations of the amount of the check.

▶ The Correct Date Is Important

- **Predating** (putting a past date on the check) is illegal.
- **Postdating** (putting a future date on the check) is also illegal. A postdated check is not good until the date listed on the check and may not be good then.

▶ Address The Check Correctly

The name of the **payee** (the person or company to whose order the check is payable) is started at the beginning of the proper line.

Titles are usually omitted. For example, a check would be written to *"John L. Carson"* (no Mr.) or *"Margaret J. Carson"* (not Mrs. John Carson).

A check written to "cash" is negotiable by anyone possessing it. Such a check can easily be stolen and cashed.

Checks written to "cash" are a weak link in expense recordkeeping and should be avoided whenever possible. (It is also preferable to avoid accepting checks made out to cash.)

▶ State The Amount Clearly

The amount of money is stated in both figures and words, and these must agree in three places:

- on the check register,
- in the figures on the right side of the check close to the dollar sign, and
- written out on the line preceding the word "dollars."

▶ Fill In The Spaces

Fill blank spaces with dashes, asterisks, or wavy lines to make it difficult to alter the amount of the check such as changing a "six " to "sixty" or raising $ 15.75 to $815.75.

► Authorized Signatures Only

Only the dentist, or another person whose signature has been formally authorized, may sign a check. Although you may be asked to write the checks, under no circumstances may you sign them <u>unless</u> yours is an authorized signature.

No matter how dire the emergency, never sign the doctor's name to a check. Doing so constitutes forgery!

► If You Make A Mistake

If a mistake is made on the check, void it and begin again. Some accountants ask that you tear the voided check across the middle or through the signature line, then tape the pieces together and save it. This way all checks can be accounted for.

► Check The Bank Balance

► Signing the doctor's name to a check is forgery!

Before sending out checks, verify the fact that the bank balance is sufficient to cover the amount involved. It is poor business to have a check returned for insufficient funds. Also, the bank will make an additional charge for handling a returned check.

COMPUTERIZED CHECK WRITING

There are computer programs available which will handle check writing, maintaining the check register, and posting expenses to the appropriate expense categories.

If the practice has a computer for accounts receivable bookkeeping and other purposes, a check writing application may also be added.

In a large practice, a more common application is to have a **payroll service** maintain computerized payroll records, prepare the payroll check and prepare the required government payroll reports.

PEGBOARD CHECK WRITING

Pegboard check writing is similar to pegboard accounting in that all records are completed in a single writing (Figs. 10-1 and 10- 4).This eliminates errors in transferring information or the hazard of forgetting to enter a check on the check register.

► The Pegboard

A pegboard, like the one used for bookkeeping, is used to position all of the necessary parts.

► The Check Register

A check register is fitted over the pegs on the left side of the board. There is a space in the middle of the form to enter deposits. The right-hand columns are used for expense catagories.

Pegboard Checks

Pegboard checks are printed with a carbonless strip across the back of the check. This strip makes it possible to write the check and the check register entry at the same time. This eliminates errors that might occur when it is necessary to make two separate data entries.

The pegboard checks come shingled in banks of twenty-five. They are positioned over the pegs so that the carbonless strip of the first check is aligned with the first available line on the check register.

Special Features

Some pegboard check writing systems include special payroll forms which make it possible to write a check and complete the payroll record at the same time.

With these systems, the payroll register is positioned between the check and the check register, and the payroll information entries are made on a special stub. The payroll register is then removed, and the check is written as usual.

How Pegboard Check Writing Works

1. The check is positioned on the check register so that the carbonless strip is over the first available line.

2. As the check is written, the information is automatically transferred by the carbonless strip from the check onto the check register.

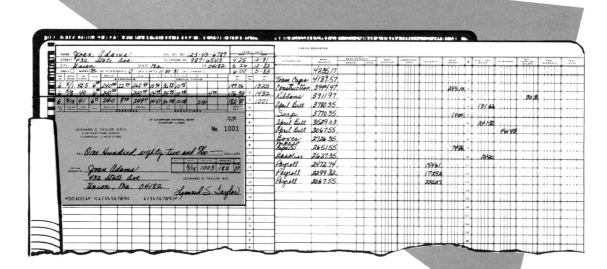

Figure 10-4. Pegboard check writing (for payroll).

3. This completes the check register entry.

4. The amount of the check should be recorded in the appropriate expense category. (This keeps expense category records up-to-date at all times.)

5. Pegboard checks fit in a double window envelope. This saves the extra step of having to address an envelope.

6. Follow the steps outlined in the Table *Verifying Pegboard Check Writing Accuracy*" to check the accuracy of your page end total and current bank balance.

VERIFYING PEGBOARD CHECK WRITING ACCURACY	
1	When starting a new page, carry forward all of the totals from the previous page. Include these figures in your calculations.
2	Total the column showing the amounts for checks written.
3	Total each expense column and record that total at the bottom of the column.
4	Add all of the expense column figures together. This number should equal the total for the "checks written" column. If it doesn't, go back and recheck your calculations. Keep looking until you have found the error.
5	In the "checks written" column, subtract the previous total (the figure at the top of the page) from the new total. The resulting number is the amount of the checks written on this page.
6	Total all deposits recorded on this page. (Be sure to include the balance forward from the previous page).
7	Subtract the amount of the checks written from the amount of the deposits. The resulting figure is the current account balance.

RECONCILING A BANK STATEMENT

It is important that the bank statement, and your check register records, be reconciled shortly after receipt of the statement. Doing this assures that your records and the bank's records are accurate and in agreement. (**Reconcile** means to settle, bring into harmony or to make consistent.)

A **bank statement** is a written accounting provided periodically by the bank. It lists all activity for that account during the statement period.

Enclosed with the statement are cancelled checks and debit memos. **Cancelled checks** are all the checks which have been paid against the account and are returned with this statement.

Debits are items, other than cancelled checks, which have been deducted directly from the account. Debits may include the service charge, returned items, or other charges. These charges are usually explained by a code at the bottom of the statement or by a **debit memorandum** enclosed with the statement.

▶ The bank statement and your checkbook records should be reconciled shortly after receipt of the statement

In order to reconcile the bank statement the following information is necessary:

- ✓ The check register
- ✓ Deposit records for the period
- ✓ The bank statement
- ✓ The accompanying cancelled checks and debit memos

THE BANK OF CHAMPAIGN

112 West Church Street

Champaign, IL 61820

Leonard S. Taylor, D.D.S.
2100 West Park Place
Champaign, IL 61820

Account Number	711-1313
Period Ending	03/10/XX
Previous Balance	$10,496.47
Ending Balance	$10,606.17

Deposits $3,864.33   **Checks** $3,756.63   **Service Charge** $5.25   **Interest Earned** $7.25

DATE	CHECK #	TRANSACTION	DEBIT	CREDIT	BALANCE
02/02/XX	479	✓ CHECK WITHDRAWAL	789.00		9,707.47
02/06/XX		✓ DEPOSIT		2,009.00	11,716.47
02/06/XX	480	✓ CHECK WITHDRAWAL	200.00		11,516.47
02/10/XX	482	✓ CHECK WITHDRAWAL	623.00		10,893.47
02/20/XX		SERVICE CHARGE	5.25		10,888.22
02/21/XX	485	✓ CHECK WITHDRAWAL	144.63		10,743.59
02/27/XX		INTEREST		7.25	10,750.84
02/27/XX		✓ DEPOSIT		1,855.33	12,606.17
02/27/XX	487	✓ CHECK WITHDRAWAL	625.75		11,980.42
02/28/XX	488	✓ CHECK WITHDRAWAL	1,374.25		10,606.17

Figure 10-5. Bank statement sample.

The Steps In Reconciling A Bank Statement

Figures 10-5 through 10-9 illustrate the data and calculations involved in reconciling a bank statement.

Step One — Verify Debits

- There should be a cancelled check or an explained debit for each charge listed on the statement.
- Compare each cancelled check with the checks listed on the statement.
- Make a mark next to the related item on the statement as it is verified against the cancelled check or debit memo.

Date	Check #	Transaction Description	Deposit	Check	Balance
		Balance Forward			$10,496.47
1/30	479✓	Robertson Supply Co.		$789.00	9,707.47
2/2	✓	deposit	$2009.00		11,716.47
2/2	480✓	Bates Answering Service		200.00	11,516.47
2/10	481	Illinois Power		326.04	11,190.43
2/10	482✓	Abbott Dental Lab		623.00	10,567.43
2/11	483	Mary Wells		257.12	10,310.31
	484	Dawson Cleaning Service		289.00	10,021.31
	485✓	Post Supply Company		144.63	9,876.68
2/20		deposit	1855.33		11,732.01
	486	petty cash		47.50	11,684.51
	487✓	Regional Dental Lab		625.75	11,058.76
	488✓	Black Realty		1374.25	9,684.51
2/28		deposit	2896.00		12,580.51

Figure 10-6. Check register sample.

174

Step Two — Verify Deposits

- Put the deposit slips in chronological order and tally deposits made against those listed on the bank statement.
- Note and make appropriate adjustments for any corrections in deposits.
- List on the worksheet by date and amount, all deposits not credited. **(Deposits Not Credited,** also referred to as **deposits in transit,** are those deposits which have been made but which were not yet credited to the account at the time of the statement.)

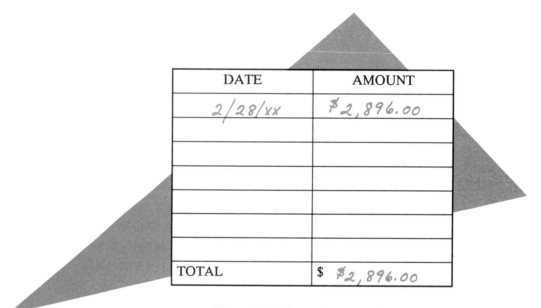

DATE	AMOUNT
2/28/xx	$2,896.00
TOTAL	$ 2,896.00

Figure 10-7. Deposits not credited.

Step Three — Verify Cancelled Checks

- Arrange the cancelled checks in numerical order and compare the cancelled checks against the check register.
- Place a mark next to the number of the cancelled check after you have determined that the amount of the check is the same as that shown on the check register.
- If a check is outstanding, circle the number of that check and list it on the worksheet by number and amount. (An **outstanding check** is any check which has been written but not yet paid by the bank.)
- When a check has been outstanding for more than three months, it may be considered lost. This check should be voided and the amount it was written for is added back to the account balance.

Step Four — Balance The Check Register

- Balance the check register through the last cancelled check or to the current date.
- Make a note in the book at the point at which it was balanced.

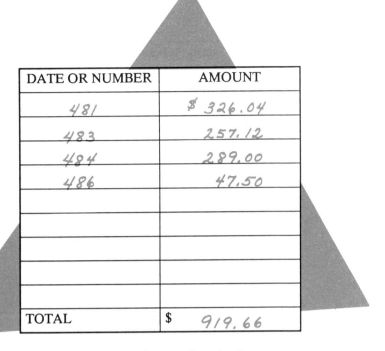

DATE OR NUMBER	AMOUNT
481	$ 326.04
483	257.12
484	289.00
486	47.50
TOTAL	$ 919.66

Figure 10-8. Outstanding checks.

Step Five — Perform The Calculations

- Follow the instructions on the worksheet and perform the necessary calculations. The two balances arrived at through these calculations should agree.
- If there are errors, they must be found and corrected. In case of bank error, it must be reported promptly.
- When the check register is reconciled with the bank statement, make a note after the last figure balanced, or draw a line under that balanced figure so that you will know where to start next month.

Step Six — Make Necessary Adjustments

- Enter all debits, such as the service charge, in the check register and deduct them from the balance.
- Also, make an entry in the check register for any interest earned on the account.

▶ If Your Account Does Not Balance

If your account does not balance, check these points carefully.

- ☐ Were <u>all</u> checks properly entered on the check register?
- ☐ Was the amount of each check entered accurately on the check register?
- ☐ Are the amounts of your deposits entered in the check register the same as those shown on your bank statement?
- ☐ Are all outstanding checks accounted for?
- ☐ Have you **added** the interest earned?

- ☐ Have you **subtracted** the service charges?
- ☐ Have all bank debit-memos been included in the check register?
- ☐ Are all worksheet calculations correct?
- ☐ Have you double checked **all** addition and subtraction in your check register?

If you are unable to reconcile the statement, contact the bank promptly and report the discrepancy.

Checkbook Information	
ENTER Balance from checkbook	$ 12,580.51
ADD Interest earned or other credits shown on statement but not in checkbook	+ 7.25
SUBTOTAL	= 12,587.76
SUBTRACT Service charge or other debits shown on statement but not in checkbook	- 5.25
CHECKBOOK BALANCE	$ 12,582.51
Bank Statement Information	
ENTER Balance from statement	$ 10,606.17
ADD Deposits not on statement	+ 2,896.00
SUBTOTAL	= 13,502.17
SUBTRACT Checks outstanding	- 919.66
STATEMENT BALANCE This balance should agree with checkbook balance	$ 12,582.51

Figure 10-9. Reconciliation calculations.

GLOSSARY

- **Abutment** - An abutment is a unit of a fixed bridge that is used to hold the pontic in place.
- **Accounts payable bookkeeping** - The management, verification, and payment of the practice expenses.
- **Accounts receivable bookkeeping** - The recording and management of all patient account transactions within the practice.
- **Accounts receivable manager** - One who is responsible for making financial arrangements with patients and for collecting all overdue accounts. Also known as *collections manager.*
- **Accounts receivable report** - A report which shows the age of accounts with an outstanding balance.
- **Adjustment** A transaction which may increase or decrease the account balance.
- **Ageing tabs** - A label which indicates the last year in which the patient was seen.
- **Anterior teeth** - The front teeth that can be seen when you smile.
- **Appointment, broken** - A scheduled appointment which the practice was not notified that the patient would be unable to keep.
- **Appointment, cancelled** - A scheduled appointment which the practice was notified that the patient would be unable to keep.
- **Appointment, changed** - Appointment times that have been filled, but which come available at the last minute because of a cancellation.
- **Appointments clerk** - One who is responsible for all scheduling of patients visits, following up on broken appointments and manage rescheduling "changed appointment" times.
- **Arch, maxillary** - See, *Maxillary arch.*
- **Arch, mandibular** - See, *Mandibular arch.*
- **Assignment of benefits** - A procedure whereby the subscriber authorizes the carrier to make payment of allowable benefits directly to the doctor.
- **Audit trail** - Records maintained to verify the integrity of the accounts receivable bookkeeping system.
- **Back order** - Notification from the supplier that a product is not available at this time.
- **Bank statement** - A written accounting provided periodically by the bank.
- **Beneficiary** - Someone who is entitled to receive benefits under an insurance plan.
- **Birthday rule** - Under coordination of benefits, the carrier for the parent who has a birthday earlier in the year is primary.
- **Bookkeeper** - One who is responsible for the management of all accounts receivable bookkeeping entries and records. The bookkeeper may also handle accounts payable bookkeeping.

- **Bridge** - A fixed appliance consisting of several units (pontics and abutments) which is used to replace missing teeth.
- **Budget plan** - An extended payment plan in which the patient has agreed to pay a certain amount each month for a fixed period of time.
- **Buffer** - A period of time saved each day to accommodate emergency patients.
- **Cancelled checks** - Checks that have been paid against the account.
- **Capitation plan** - An HMO plan under which the dentists are paid a flat fee for each patient under the practice's care, regardless of the amount of care actually provided.
- **Carrier** - An insurance company which agrees to pay benefits claimed under a health plan.
- **Carrier, primary** - Under coordination of benefits, the carrier who is responsible to pay first the benefits that the beneficiary is entitled to receive.
- **Carrier, secondary** - Under coordination of benefits, the carrier who is responsible to pay at least a portion of the balance after the primary carrier has made payment.
- **Cash policy** - A payment plan requesting that all fees be paid, in full, at the time of treatment.
- **Cash discount** - A reduction in the amount owed if the amount of the proposed treatment plan is paid in full before treatment begins.
- **Cash policy, modified** - See, *Monthly statements.*
- **Cavity classifications** - A system of identifying and describing types of locations of cavities and restorations.
- **Change fund** - A limited amount of cash kept for the purpose of making change for patients paying cash.
- **Charge slip** - A form used to transmit account information from the business office to the treatment area and back again to the business office. Also known as a *superbill, encounter form, routing slip,* or *transmittal document.*
- **Charge** - A transaction which increases the account balance.
- **Chart, patient** - Those clinical records for a patient which are stored together.
- **Child** - For purposes of defining dependent eligibility, a dependent who does not exceed the age as designated in the contract.
- **Civilian Health and Medical Program of the Uniformed Services (CHAMPUS)** - A federal program designed to provide eligible beneficiaries a supplement to medical care in military and Public Health Service facilities.
- **Claim form** - A format used for reporting the information necessary for the processing of an insurance claim.
- **Coinsurance** - A provision of a program by which the beneficiary shares in the cost of covered expenses on a percentage basis.
- **Copayment** - See, *Coinsurance.*

- **Collection agency** - A company which specializes in collecting overdue accounts.
- **Consummables** - Supplies and minor pieces of equipment which are used up fairly quickly.
- **Coordination of benefits** - When covered by more than one group plan, the patient may not receive payment from both carriers that comes to more than 100% of the actual expenses.
- **Crown** - A cast restoration which covers the entire anatomic crown of a tooth.
- **Customary fee** - The fee for a given service is set by the carrier. The carrier sets the customary fee at a percentile of the usual fees charged by doctors with similar training and experience within the same geographic area.
- **Cycle billing** - A system of preparing statements in which statements are sent to different parts of the alphabet throughout the month.
- **Daily schedule** - A printed list of all patients scheduled for the day which is posted in key areas of the office.
- **Daily journal** - A record of all charges, payments and adjustments to the bookkeeping system made on a daily basis.
- **Debits** - Items, other than cancelled checks, that have been deducted from the account.
- **Deductible** - A stipulated amount that the covered person must pay toward the cost of care before the benefits of the program go into effect.
- **Defendant** - The person being called into court.
- **Dentition** - The natural teeth in the dental arch.
- **Dentition, primary** - The first 20 teeth to erupt which are shed naturally. Also known as *baby* or *milk teeth.*
- **Dentition, permanent** - The thirty-two teeth which are designed to last a lifetime.
- **Denture, partial** - An appliance used to replace some missing teeth in an arch.
- **Denture, full** - An appliance used to replace all of the teeth in an edentulous arch.
- **Deposits not credited** - Deposits which have been made but are not yet credited to the account.
- **Deposits in transit** - See, *Deposits not credited.*
- **Depreciation** - The process of writing off the cost of major equipment purchases.
- **Distal** - Away from the midline.
- **Divided payment plan** - A payment plan in which the timing of two or three payments is based on the stage of treatment.
- **Down-coding** - The practice of reimbursing according to the lowest paying code that fits the description given.
- **Dual coverage** - Insurance coverage for an individual provided under more than one group plan.

- **Edentulous** means without teeth, and refers to having lost all of the natural teeth.
- **Electronic Claims** - The transmission of insurance claims from one computer to another.
- **Eligibility** - The right of an individual to receive benefits under a specific plan.
- **Embezzlement** - The illegal act of stealing practice funds by manipulating the bookkeeping records.
- **Endodontist** - A dental specialist who treats diseases and injuries of the dental pulp.
- **Estimate form** - A form used to present to the patient a written estimate of the cost of the proposed treatment plan.
- **Exclusions** - Specific services which are not covered by a plan.
- **Facial** - Toward the lips and cheek.
- **Fair Credit Reporting Act** - A Federal law concerning the reporting of credit ratings.
- **Fee, customary** - See, *Customary fee.*
- **Fee, usual** - See, *Usual fee.*
- **Fee-for-service** - A payment system, under which the doctor is paid on the basis of services actually rendered.
- **FICA** - Federal Insurance Contributions Act. See also, *Social Security.*
- **File clerk** - One who is responsible for filing and retrieving patient records as needed.
- **File, drawer** - Records are stored and protected in file drawers. Also known as *vertical files.*
- **File, lateral** - Records are stored and protected on shelves. Also known as *open shelf filing.*
- **File guide** - A divider used to improve the organization of files.
- **File guide, auxiliary** - A divider that establishes a subheading within a primary guide.
- **File guide, primary** - A divider used for the main subject, letter of the alphabet or numerical headings.
- **Filing, alphabetical** - The organization and storage of records in alphabetical order.
- **Filing chronological** - The organization and storage of records in order by date.
- **Filing, cross-reference** - A file which is maintained in alphabetical order to make it possible to locate materials which have been filed numerically.
- **Filing, numerical** - The organization and storage of records in numerical order.
- **Filing, subject** - The organization of records by topic. The subjects are then filed alphabetically.
- **Finance charge** - An additional charge which is added to an overdue account.

- **Fixed prosthetics** - The replacement of missing teeth with an appliance that is cemented in place and cannot be removed by the patient. Also known as *crown and bridge.*
- **FUTA** - Federal Unemployment Tax.
- **Given name** - See, *Name, given.*
- **Gross pay** - The amount earned before taxes are deducted.
- **Guide, out** - See, *Out guide.*
- **Health maintenance organization** (HMO) - A health care delivery system in which a flat monthly premium is paid to the HMO to provide necessary health care services for the patient (as specified in the contract).
- **Holidays, minor** - Those holidays when schools and some businesses are closed, but the office is open.
- **Holidays, major** - Those holidays when the office is closed.
- **Incisal** - Biting edge.
- **Independent practice association** (IPA) - A type of HMO formed and run by dentists who enter into agreements to provide dental services to a defined group of persons.
- **Indexing** - The process of determining the order in which the units of a name are to be considered.
- **Insurance clerk** - One who is responsible for completing, filing and following-up on all insurance claims and payments.
- **Insured** - The person who represents the family unit in relation to the insurance plan.
- **Interproximal** - Between the teeth.
- **Invoice** - An itemized list of goods shipped which includes pricing information.
- **Judgement** - A court order stating that the defendant must pay the monies owed.
- **Jurisdiction** - The location in which a case must be tried.
- **Lead time** - The time lapse between ordering and receiving the product.
- **Ledger card** - A paper form used to record account history data in a manual bookkeeping system.
- **Lingual** - Toward the tongue.
- **Maiden name** - See, *Name, maiden.*
- **Malocclusion** - When the teeth are not positioned in the proper relationship to each other.
- **Mandibular arch** - The lower jaw.
- **Matrixing** - Establishing the format of the appointment book. Also known as *outlining.*
- **Maxillary arch** - The upper jaw.
- **Maximums** - Limitations on payments for specific services. These may be annual maximums or lifetime maximums.
- **Medicaid** - A government program to provide health and dental care for the poor.

- **Medical and dental history** - A form used to gather and organize data concerning the patient's past and current medical and dental history.
- **Medicare** - A federal government program to provide health care for the elderly.
- **Mesial** - Toward the midline.
- **Modem** - A telephone line link between computers.
- **N.S.F. check** - A check returned by the bank because there were not sufficient funds in the account to pay the amount of the check.
- **Name, given** - An individual's first name
- **Name, last** - See, *Surname.*
- **Name, maiden** - A woman's surname before she marries.
- **Net pay** - The amount received after deductions have been subtracted.
- **Noncapitation plan** - An HMO plan under which the doctors are paid according to the number of patients they see over a given period of time.
- **Occlusal** - The chewing surfaces.
- **Office manager** - One who is responsible for the supervision of all business office activities.
- **Oral surgeon** - A dental specialist who specializes in the surgical treatment of diseases, injuries, and defects involving the teeth and the hard and soft tissues of the oral and maxillofacial regions.
- **Order quantity** - The optimal amount of a given item to be purchased at one time.
- **Orthodontist** - A dental specialist concerned with the correction of all forms of malocclusion.
- **Out guide** - A marker used in the filing system to indicate where a file folder has been removed.
- **Outlining** - See, *Matrixing.*
- **Outstanding check** - A check that has been written but not yet paid by the bank.
- **Overhead** - Those expenses which represent the dentist's cost of doing business.
- **Packing slip** - An itemized list of goods shipped. It does not contain pricing information.
- **Patient Registration form** - A form used to gather primarily financial data concerning the person responsible for the account.
- **Payee** - The person to whom the check is written.
- **Payment** - A transaction which decreases the account balance.
- **Payor** - The person writing the check.
- **Pediatric dentist** - A dental specialist concerned with treating children from birth through adolescence.
- **Periodontist** - A dental specialist concerned with the diagnosis and treatment of disease of the tissues which surround and support the teeth.
- **Permanent dentition** - Dentition, permanent.
- **Petty cash** - A limited amount of cash kept in the office to pay small expenses.

- **Plaintiff** - The person who has brought the case to court.
- **Plan** - An insurance contract which the carrier has written to provide specific benefits to those covered by the plan.
- **Pontic** - A unit of the bridge which is used to replace a missing tooth.
- **Postdating** - Putting a future date on a check.
- **Posterior teeth** - The back teeth that are used for chewing.
- **Posting** - The act of entering transaction information into the bookkeeping system.
- **Predating** - Putting a past date on a check.
- **Preferred provider organization** (PPO) - A formal agreement among health care providers to treat a specific patient population at an agreed upon rate.
- **Primary carrier** - See, *Carrier, primary.*
- **Primary dentition** - See *Dentition, primary.*
- **Prosthodontist** - A dental specialist concerned with in the replacement of missing teeth.
- **Purchase order** - A form authorizing the purchase of specific supplies from a specific supplier.
- **Purge tabs** - See, *Ageing tabs.*
- **Quadrant** - One of four sections.
- **Question, closed-ended** - A question that can be answered "yes" or "no."
- **Question, open-ended** - A question which requires more than a "yes" or "no" answer.
- **Rapport** - A feeling of harmony and accord.
- **Receipt** - A form given to the patient to acknowledge a cash payment. Also used to inform the patient of the current account balance.
- **Receptionist** - One who is responsible for answering the telephones, greeting practice visitors, typing and correspondence, and the smooth functioning of the reception area.
- **Reconcile** - To settle, bring into harmony. To verify the balance of the bank statement against that of the check register.
- **Red flag reorder tag** - A paper tag used to mark the reorder point of a supply.
- **Referral source** - The name of the person or source which referred the new patient to the practice.
- **Release of Information** - The patient's signature giving the doctor permission to release information regarding the patient's condition and treatment.
- **Removable prosthetics** - The replacement of missing teeth with an appliance that can be placed and removed by the patient.
- **Reorder point** - The minimum quantity of a given item which is an adequate reserve for that product.
- **Restrictive endorsement** - An endorsement placed on the back of a check to prevent it from being cashed if stolen.

- **Routing guide** - Guidelines, provided by the dentist, as to how different types of phone calls are to be handled.
- **Schedule of benefits** - A specified amount which the carrier will pay toward the cost of covered health services.
- **Secondary carrier** - See, *Carrier secondary.*
- **Secondary address** - The name and address of the nearest relative <u>not</u> living with the person completing the registration form.
- **Shelf life** - The length of time that an item may be kept in stock before it deteriorates and loses its effectiveness.
- **Signature on file** - The patient's signature on record authorizing the release of information and/or the assignment of benefits.
- **Skip tracing** - Efforts to find a debtor who has moved without leaving a forwarding address.
- **Small claims court** - A court which handles only claims for small amounts of monies owed.
- **Social Security** - A federal payroll tax in which the employer makes a matching contribution.
- **Spouse** - The wife or husband of the insured.
- **Statements** - A notice sent to inform the responsible party of the amount of the outstanding balance due on the account.
- **Stop payment order** - An order to the bank to stop payment on a check.
- **Subscriber** - See, *Insured.*
- **Superbill** - A form that is used to simplify reporting treatment information in the office and/or on an insurance claim form.
- **Surname** - Last name
- **Teeth, anterior** - See, *Anterior teeth.*
- **Teeth, posterior** - See, *Posterior teeth.*
- **Term denoting seniority** - Jr., Sr., or a Roman numeral.
- **Transaction** - Any financial entry made to an account record.
- **Treatment plan** - The dentist's recommendations for treatment which are based on the examination findings.
- **Truth In Lending** - A Federal law concerning extended payment plans which requires disclosure if there is a finance charge or if there are four or more payments with or without a finance charge.
- **Universal Numbering System** - The system adopted by the American Dental Association to assure accuracy in identification of the teeth.
- **Usual fee** - The fee that is usually charged, for a given service, by a dentist to private practice.
- **Wage and tax statement** (W-2) - The form which shows total earnings and taxes withheld for the calender year.
- **Walk-in** - An individual, without an appointment, who comes to the practice seeking care.
- **Walk-out statement** - A form used to inform the patient of the current account balance and to encourage prompt payment.

- **Welcome brochure** - A brochure given to a new patient to provide information about the practice.
- **Withholding exemption certificate** (W-4) - A form on which the employee indicates the number of exemptions claimed for tax purposes.
- **Work-in** - A patient requiring only a brief visit which can be worked into another patient's scheduled time.
- **Workers' compensation** - A state program to cover the medical expenses for employees who are injured on the job.

Index